Studies in Applied Philosophy, Epistemology and Rational Ethics

Volume 58

Editor-in-Chief

Lorenzo Magnani, Department of Humanities, Philosophy Section, University of Pavia, Pavia, Italy

Editorial Board

Atocha Aliseda
Universidad Nacional Autónoma de México (UNAM), Mexico, Mexico

Giuseppe Longo
CNRS - Ecole Normale Supérieure, Centre Cavailles, Paris, France

Chris Sinha
School of Foreign Languages, Hunan University, Changsha, China

Paul Thagard
University of Waterloo, Waterloo, Canada

John Woods
University of British Columbia, Vancouver, Canada

Studies in Applied Philosophy, Epistemology and Rational Ethics (SAPERE) publishes new developments and advances in all the fields of philosophy, epistemology, and ethics, bringing them together with a cluster of scientific disciplines and technological outcomes: ranging from computer science to life sciences, from economics, law, and education to engineering, logic, and mathematics, from medicine to physics, human sciences, and politics. The series aims at covering all the challenging philosophical and ethical themes of contemporary society, making them appropriately applicable to contemporary theoretical and practical problems, impasses, controversies, and conflicts. Our scientific and technological era has offered "new" topics to all areas of philosophy and ethics – for instance concerning scientific rationality, creativity, human and artificial intelligence, social and folk epistemology, ordinary reasoning, cognitive niches and cultural evolution, ecological crisis, ecologically situated rationality, consciousness, freedom and responsibility, human identity and uniqueness, cooperation, altruism, intersubjectivity and empathy, spirituality, violence. The impact of such topics has been mainly undermined by contemporary cultural settings, whereas they should increase the demand of interdisciplinary applied knowledge and fresh and original understanding. In turn, traditional philosophical and ethical themes have been profoundly affected and transformed as well: they should be further examined as embedded and applied within their scientific and technological environments so to update their received and often old-fashioned disciplinary treatment and appeal. Applying philosophy individuates therefore a new research commitment for the 21st century, focused on the main problems of recent methodological, logical, epistemological, and cognitive aspects of modeling activities employed both in intellectual and scientific discovery, and in technological innovation, including the computational tools intertwined with such practices, to understand them in a wide and integrated perspective. **Studies in Applied Philosophy, Epistemology and Rational Ethics** means to demonstrate the contemporary practical relevance of this novel philosophical approach and thus to provide a home for monographs, lecture notes, selected contributions from specialized conferences and workshops as well as selected Ph.D. theses. The series welcomes contributions from philosophers as well as from scientists, engineers, and intellectuals interested in showing how applying philosophy can increase knowledge about our current world. Initial proposals can be sent to the Editor-in-Chief, Prof. Lorenzo Magnani, lmagnani@unipv.it:

- A short synopsis of the work or the introduction chapter
- The proposed Table of Contents
- The CV of the lead author(s).

For more information, please contact the Editor-in-Chief at lmagnani@unipv.it.

Indexed by SCOPUS, ISI and Springerlink. The books of the series are submitted for indexing to Web of Science.

More information about this series at http://www.springer.com/series/10087

Daniele Chiffi

Clinical Reasoning: Knowledge, Uncertainty, and Values in Health Care

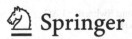 Springer

Daniele Chiffi
DAStU
Politecnico di Milano
Milan, Italy

ISSN 2192-6255   ISSN 2192-6263 (electronic)
Studies in Applied Philosophy, Epistemology and Rational Ethics
ISBN 978-3-030-59096-3   ISBN 978-3-030-59094-9 (eBook)
https://doi.org/10.1007/978-3-030-59094-9

This Springer imprint is published by the registered company Springer Nature Switzerland AG
The registered company address is: Gewerbestrasse 11, 6330 Cham, Switzerland

To Elsa

Acknowledgements

I am grateful to many colleagues and friends for their helpful suggestions and discussions: Ahti-Veikko Pietarinen, Massimiliano Carrara, Lorenzo Magnani, John Woods, Giovanni Boniolo, Paola Berchialla, Dario Gregori, Ciro De Florio, Fabrizio Macagno, Mario Castellana, Ileana Baldi, Pierdaniele Giaretta, Renzo Zanotti, Annalisa Malara, Erich Rast, Ingvar Johansson, Donald E. Stanley, Cristina Canova, Francesca Foltran, Simonetta Ballali, Ari Voutilainen, Alexander Hochdorn, Mattia Andreoletti, Giuseppe Primiero, Behnam Taebi, Matthieu Fontaine, Cristina Barés Gómez, Selene Arfini, Piera Poletti, Alessandro Grecucci, Francesca Foltran, Maria Grazia Rossi, Pekka Louhiala, Dina Mendonça, Barbara Osimani, Raffaella Campaner, Federica Russo, Alessandro Pagnini, Cristina Amoretti, Federico Boem, Marco Annoni, and all my co-authors.

Moreover, I wish to acknowledge some people for their more or less tangible help: Francesco Bellucci, Damiano Canale, Giovanni Tuzet, Marta Pozza, Egle Perissinotto, Gabriele Biandolino, Roberto Ciuni, Pietro Gori, Fabien Schang, David Dueñas-Cid, Giovanni D'oria, Giacomo Signore, Alfredo Di Giorgio, Jelena Issajeva, Marika Proover, Fabio Ciracì, Amirouche Moktefi, Vittorio Morato, Javier González de Prado Salas, Martin Stokhof, Michiel van Lambalgen, Aldo Frigerio, Paolo Stellino, Gianluca Caterina, Rocco Gangle, Fabio Minazzi, Vincenzo Fano, Jan Sprenger, Roberto Giuntini, Carlo Martini, Federico Laudisa, Gustavo Cevolani, Edoardo Datteri, Giovani Carrozzini, Caterina Annese, Massimo Bricocoli, Gabriele Pasqui, Sandro Balducci, Stefano Moroni, Francesco Curci, Paolo Beria, Agostino Petrillo, Costanzo Ranci, Alessandra Oppio, and all colleagues at DAStU (Politecnico di Milano).

I need to express a great deal of gratitude to the "dream team" of META (Social Sciences and Humanities for Science and Technology) Unit at Politecnico di Milano, namely Simona Chiodo, Viola Schiaffonati, Paolo Volontè, Giovanni Valente, Stefano Crabu, Fabio Fossa, and Paolo Bory.

Claudia Ampuero greatly helped me to further improve the style of the text. Leontina Di Cecco and Monica Janet Michael contributed significantly to an efficient book production.

A special thanks goes to Orazio, Cristina, and Chiara for their continuous support.

Finally, two anonymous reviewers provided me with many thoughtful suggestions and remarks, which helped me improve some of the arguments discussed in the book.

This book is the result of more than 10 years of research in clinical reasoning conducted in the following European research institutions:

- Unit of Biostatistics, Epidemiology and Public Health (University of Padova)
- Unit of Nursing Studies (University of Padova)
- Group of Philosophy of Science and Technology—Ragnar Nurkse Department of Innovation and Governance (Tallinn University of Technology)
- IFILNOVA, Reasoning and Argumentation Laboratory (ARGLAB), New University of Lisbon
- DAStU, Politecnico di Milano.

Over the last decade, the following grants have sustained the work on the present book (in chronological order): *Economic Impact of High Cost Drugs in the Veneto Region*, Research Project Agreement, University of Padova (2010–2012); *Decision Making and Argumentation in Medicine and Nursing Theory* (grant project/University of Padova, 2013–2014); *Rules of logical-probabilistic formalization of hypothetical reasoning in clinical nursing*, University of Padova, Research Grant (2014–2016); *Abduction in the Age of Fundamental Uncertainty*—PUT1305—Estonian Research Council—ERC (2016–2018); *Hypothetical Reasoning*, Erasmus+ project, University of Padova (2018); *Values in Argumentative Discourse*, Project PTDC/MHC-FIL/0521/2014 of the Portuguese Fundação para a Ciência e a Tecnologia, (2018–2019); Excellence Program *Fragilità Territoriali*, DAStU—Politecnico di Milano, funded by the Italian Ministry of Education (2018–2022; L. 232/2016).

I am grateful to Springer for permission to include (portions of) previously published papers and to Oxford University Press, Wiley Blackwell, and the journals listed below for agreeing to insert in this book deeply modified and updated versions of my papers. The list of original publications is the following:

Chiffi, D., Zanotti, R.: Medical and nursing diagnoses: a critical comparison. Journal of evaluation in clinical practice **21**(1), 1–6 (2015).
Zanotti, R., Chiffi, D.: Diagnostic frameworks and nursing diagnoses: a normative stance. Nursing Philosophy **16**(1), 64–73 (2015).
Giaretta, P., Chiffi, D.: Varieties of Probability in Clinical Diagnosis. Acta Baltica Historiae et Philosophiae Scientiarum **6**(1), 5–27 (2018).
Chiffi, D., Zanotti, R.: Fear of knowledge: clinical hypotheses in diagnostic and prognostic reasoning. Journal of evaluation in clinical practice **23**(5), 928–934 (2017).
Chiffi, D., Andreoletti, M.: What's Going to Happen to Me? Prognosis in the Face of Uncertainty. Topoi, 1–8, doi: 10.1007/s11245-019-09684-z (2019).

Chiffi, D., Zanotti, R.: Perspectives on clinical possibility: elements of analysis. Journal of evaluation in clinical practice **22**(4), 509–514 (2016).

Chiffi, D., Zanotti, R.: Knowledge and belief in placebo effect. The Journal of Medicine and Philosophy: A Forum for Bioethics and Philosophy of Medicine **42** (1), 70–85 (2017).

Zanotti, R., Chiffi, D.: Nursing knowledge: hints from the placebo effect. Nursing Philosophy **18**(3), e12140 (2017).

Zanotti, R., Chiffi, D.: A normative analysis of nursing knowledge. Nursing inquiry **23**(1), 4–11 (2016).

Chiffi, D., Pietarinen, A.-V.: Clinical equipoise and moral leeway: An epistemological stance. Topoi **38**, 447–456 (2019).

Chiffi, D., Foltran, F., Gregori, D.: Dealing with the complexity of health-related risk communication: philosophical and cognitive aspects behind "informed consent" within a person-centered context. International Journal of Person Centered Medicine **1**(3), 494–500 (2011).

Contents

Chapter 1
Introduction

The book is intended to shed new light on the classical themes of philosophy of clinical disciplines (e.g. the nature of diagnosis, prognosis, placebo effect, etc.), in particular on those involved in the theoretical foundations of medical practice and nursing theory.

Contemporary literature in clinical reasoning and philosophy of medicine is for the most part focused on the role of big data in the health context; however, an attempt to provide any deep reflection of the logical structure of clinical reasoning seems to be lacking.

This book is geared towards bridging such gap by breaking down the logical and clinical components of medical reasoning in which the 'small data' of signs, symptoms and medical hypotheses may have a considerable impact on the way clinicians (i) think and formulate their judgments, (ii) substantiate clinical knowledge and (iii) provide care to patients and communicate with them.

Another seminal feature of the book is the analysis of severe forms of uncertainty (and even ignorance), which may permeate the foundations of clinical reasoning and practice. Despite the immense biostatistical literature, I think there is still room for an abductive methodology to be applied in the health context in order to deal in particular with severe forms of clinical uncertainty.

Finally, the book investigates the normative facets of clinical knowledge and the interplay between biomedical knowledge, clinical practice, and research and values. In bioethics, it is quite common to only investigate the ethical values associated to medicine. This book, instead, attempts to interpret the difficult interaction between epistemic and non-epistemic aspects of values and clinical knowledge, with a special emphasis on nursing knowledge, whose aims and methods go beyond the biomedical model of care.

For those who want to gain a thorough and cumulative understanding of the treated issues, the book can be read in its entirety; though, each chapter may be also read

D. Chiffi, *Clinical Reasoning: Knowledge, Uncertainty, and Values in Health Care*, Studies in Applied Philosophy, Epistemology and Rational Ethics 58, https://doi.org/10.1007/978-3-030-59094-9_1

independently of one another to concentrate on a specific aspect of clinical reasoning. Differing from previous literature on the topic, *a clear philosophical emphasis* is here provided on themes and methods that are at the crossing between diverse disciplines: medicine, nursing, logic, epistemology, philosophy of science, ethics, epidemiology, and statistics. For instance, it is not uncommon that in books devoted to clinical thinking the word "philosophy" can be even absent. See, for instance, (Del Mar et al. 2006).

Beyond a clear philosophical emphasis, the present book is particularly sensitive to different professional approaches to clinical practice. Indeed, even among clinical disciplines, I will provide many reasons to show, for instance, how the reasoning patterns of medical doctors may be methodologically different from the ones used by nurses and other clinical professionals, notwithstanding, of course, the need to acknowledge a common ground between these actors. In fact, I do not fully endorse the view that for all kinds of clinical professionals "the rules of the game are same. [They] all share the same ways of thinking" (Jenicek 2012, xxx). I prefer to say, using Wittgensteinian terminology, that there are similar, but different games showing a family resemblance. Clinical reasoning calls for critical reflections on health and disease in a specific clinical context, which touches upon the methods and resources of many different clinical and non-clinical disciplines forming a unified framework. This shows the interdisciplinary nature of clinical reasoning, which may be greatly shaped by nursing knowledge and practice. The present book intends to fill this gap also because, even in remarkable works devoted to clinical reasoning such as (Mongtomery 2005), the issues of nursing knowledge, theory and practice have been—as explicitly stated by the author—considerably overlooked.[1]

Therefore, in the effort to propose an integrative approach to health and disease, I will engage in a deep analysis of different forms of clinical judgments involved in the notions of diagnosis, prognosis, treatment, placebo effect, and so forth. Moreover, a thorough philosophical investigation on the values involved in health care is provided, based on clinical and philosophical literature.

New forms of clinical reasoning sensitive to clinical practice are investigated providing a rigorous logical ground for clinical reasoning, with a special emphasis on abductive modes of reasoning. Nonetheless, classical statistical and probabilistic issues in health care are also considered in a philosophical nuance. On the one hand, the book offers an investigation of some theoretical limitations and potential amendments of Evidence Based Medicine. On the other hand, it proposes a fresh view on nursing knowledge and practice. The main idea is to treat health and disease from a philosophical perspective that takes into consideration all health care professionals, overcoming the limitations of the so-called "classical biomedical model of care". The lines of thought of my approach to health care will be mainly guided by an assessment of the role of uncertainty in clinical research and practice and through a critical reflection on (moral) argumentation in health care.

---

[1]For a comprehensive view on clinical reasoning in different health professions, see (Higgs et al. 2019).

The final phase of the making of this book has coincided with the outbreak of Covid-19 pandemic while I was in Milan, Lombardy (Italy), one of the most affected regions in the world. Thus, as is evident from the lines below, sound clinical reasoning in health care is also crucial to managing health care crises of this magnitude.

1.1 Clinical Reasoning and the Outbreak of the Covid-19 Pandemic: The Diagnosis of the So-Called "Patient 1" in Italy

Annalisa Malara, 38 years old, an anaesthesiologist from Cremona (Lombardy, Italy) who works in Codogno hospital is said to have "changed everyone's life in Italy".[2] On 21 February 2020, she was the first Italian doctor to diagnose the Covid-19 disease in a patient (who did not have any known connection with China) in the country, prompting for the clinical protocol for suspected Covid-19 cases. The patient, named Mattia Maestri, was a 38-year-old researcher who—as reported by local newspapers—practiced sports and had no previous medical history of such disease. An example of the protocol that was used before the diagnosis of Mattia is, for instance, the one created by the Italian Society for Infectious and Tropical Diseases (SIMIT).[3] This protocol was composed by three types of criteria: an epidemiological, a clinical and a temporal criterion (the well-known 14 days of incubation of Covid-19 disease); moreover, it was organized as a flow chart. The first criterion that had to go under scrutiny was the epidemiological one; it required to test for Covid-19 whether the patient (i) would have been in regions at risk (during that time mainly China), (ii) would have had previous professional or non-professional close contacts with probable or confirmed cases affected by Covid-19, and (iii) would have declared professional or non-professional attendance at hospitals where patients were treated for Covid-19. If at least one of the conditions (i–iii) was met, then the protocol allowed medical doctors and nurses to consider the subsequent clinical and temporal criteria in order to decide for possible hospitalization of the patient. If, however, no conditions for the epidemiological criterion was fulfilled, then the protocol suggested excluding the possibility of the patient being a case of Covid-19, and not incurring in the evaluation of the remaining criteria. This taxonomical way of reasoning was maybe too rigid and non-optimal given the (unknown) local diffusion of the disease in the Italian population.

---

[2]La dottoressa di Codogno che ha scoperto il "paziente uno": «Sono andata oltre la prassi e ho cercato l'impossibile», *Open*, 6 March 2020, https://www.open.online/2020/03/06/la-dottoressa-di-codogno-che-ha-scoperto-il-paziente-uno-ho-cercato-impossibile/ .

[3]Gestione del sospetto caso di Infezione da 2019-nCoV da parte del personale sanitario in Ospedale (PS e altri reparti) e Territorio—Scheda 1, versione 3.0—04/02/2020. https://www.infermieristica mente.it/articolo/11373/coronavirus:-ecco-le-linee-guida-operative-e-gestionali-della-simit-(sca ricabili-nell-articolo). However, doctor Malara confirmed me that in Codogno hospital a slightly different protocol for suspected cases of Covid-19 patients was used.

The first time Mattia went to the emergency room at the hospital in Codogno for a mild pneumonia, no hospitalization was suggested to him since the epidemiological criterion was not fulfilled. However, he went back to the hospital some days later since his lung infection was not responding to any known standard treatment. And it was at his point that Annalisa Malara pushed forward the clinical hypothesis of Mattia having contracted Covid-19. As we will see, this is one form of abductive reasoning, a crucial ingredient of clinical reasoning as we will see in the book. Malara stated that "for the first time, drugs and treatments were ineffective on an apparently trivial pneumonia. My duty was to heal that sick person. By exclusion, I concluded that if the known failed, all I had to do was enter the unknown. The coronavirus was hiding right here,"[4] and she added "When a patient does not respond to normal treatment, at university they taught me not to ignore the worst hypothesis".[5] After a few hours, a laboratory test would result in Mattia becoming "patient 1" in Italy, and Annalisa Malara as the doctor who identified the Italian outbreak (the first one in the Western world). Then, an epidemiological investigation in the form of retrospective (abductive) reasoning was carried out in order to trace the people that had come in contact with Mattia, who were unfortunately many since he had attended a lot of sport events some days prior to the diagnosis (including running races and football matches in different areas of Northern Italy).

Thus, thanks to the clinical acumen of Malara, the whole country could start fighting against Covid-19. A month after, Mattia was discharged from the hospital, his father passed away because of Covid-19 and he became a father some weeks later.

I think that the Italian "Patient 1" story shows the (i) *interplay between known and unknown factors* in clinical reasoning, (ii) the methodological and clinical problems of *uncritically relying on fixed taxonomical procedures and protocols* that may be based on incorrect assumptions, (iii) the deep sense of *moral duty* that the anaesthesiologist felt towards the patient, and (iv) the cogency of assuming correct *forms of clinical reasoning*, in particular for abductive inferences connecting biomedical knowledge with the signs and symptoms of the patient. All these factors are key elements of the present book. This vivid example puts into perspective just how clinical knowledge can be enhanced and uncertainty mitigated when using correct forms of reasoning in health care.

---

[4] *Ibidem.*

[5] G. Visetti, Coronavirus, l'anestesista di Codogno che ha intuito la diagnosi di Mattia: "Ho pensato all'impossibile", Repubblica, 6 March 2020, https://www.repubblica.it/cronaca/2020/03/06/news/l_anestesista_di_codogno_per_mattia_era_tutto_inutile_cosi_ho_avuto_la_folle_idea_di_pensare_al_coronavirus_-250380291/ .

1.2 The Content of the Book

The book is composed by two parts and 13 chapters. Part I, *Clinical Judgment*, includes Chaps. 2–5 and addresses the foundations of clinical judgments, in particular regarding diagnostic and prognostic processes. Part II, *Philosophy of Clinical Reasoning, Research and Practice*, includes Chaps. 6–14 and provides an analysis of some relevant notions in clinical reasoning such as clinical possibility, nursing knowledge, values in health care, clinical equipoise and informed consent, among others.

Chapter 2, *Foundations of Clinical Diagnosis*, presents the logical structure of clinical diagnosis by making a comparison between clinical medicine and nursing. Then, diagnostic frameworks are investigated in light of their normative, temporal and teleological components.

Chapter 3, *Probability in Clinical Diagnosis*, analyses the crossing-over of different types of probability involved in making the diagnostic judgment. As such, varied scenarios associated to realistic clinical cases are discussed and critically evaluated.

Chapter 4, *Clinical Hypotheses in Diagnostic and Prognostic Reasoning*, points out the role of clinical hypotheses for the justification of diagnostic and prognostic judgments. Moreover, a deep analysis is made of the viability of abductive inference for clinical reasoning in presence of fundamental uncertainty.

Chapter 5, *Prognosis in the Face of Uncertainty*, focuses on the role of fundamental uncertainty for prognostication, and shows the limitations of providing a fixed explication of the notion of prognostic judgment merely based on the biomedical model.

Chapter 6, *On Clinical Possibility*, proposes a critical reflection on the notion of clinical possibility. Although such concept is extensively used in clinical reasoning, no thorough examination has been provided so far of what exactly is meant by clinical possibility. Starting from some relevant features associated with the concept, I argue that almost all clinical possibilities are potentialities, i.e. possibilities that may be actualised by effective, appropriate and feasible interventions.

Chapter 7, *The Epistemology of Placebo Effect*, is about the alleged self-fulfilling nature of placebo beliefs. Many epistemologists focused on the self-fulfilling nature of these beliefs, which have raised some important counterexamples to Nozick's "tracking theory of knowledge". In this chapter, I challenge this particularity of placebo-based beliefs in multi-agent contexts, by analysing their deep epistemological nature and the role of higher-order beliefs involved in the placebo effect.

Chapter 8, *Nursing Knowledge and Placebo Effect*, analyses the placebo effect in the clinical practice of nursing. Such effect may be a powerful tool in nursing and may clarify its disciplinary knowledge compared to the classical biomedical model of health care.

Chapter 9, *Nursing Knowledge and Values*, addresses the question of normative analysis of the value-based aspects of nursing. By analysing the roles of the various forms of (epistemic and non-epistemic) values and models of knowledge translation, a better comprehension of the specific role of values in nursing can be reached. A conceptual framework has been built to classify some of the classical perspectives on nursing knowledge and to examine the relationships between values and different forms of knowledge in nursing.

Chapter 10, *Clinical Equipoise and Moral Leeway*, investigates the principle of clinical equipoise, which has been proposed as an ethical tool relating uncertainty and moral permissibility in clinical research. This chapter presents a new argument that brings out the epistemological difficulties we encounter in justifying clinical equipoise in medical research.

Chapter 11, *Philosophical and Cognitive Elements of Risk Communication in Informed Consent*, addresses the interplay between health risk perception and communication. This chapter argues that the effectiveness of risk communication in the health domain can be greatly improved by considering the cognitive and emotional biases involved and all the factors affecting risk perception.

Chapter 12, *Concluding Thoughts: Towards a Clinical Philosophy*, points out new lines of research for shaping clinical reasoning in the current age of technology and uncertainty.

Appendix, *The Diagnosis of Covid-19 for "Patient 1" in Italy* concludes the book.

References

Del Mar, C., Doust, J., Glasziou, P.: Clinical Thinking Communication and Decision-Making. . Blackwell Publishing Inc., , Malden (2006)

Higgs, J., Jones, M.A., Loftus, S., Christensen, N. (eds.).: Clinical Reasoning in the Health Professions, 4th edn. Elsevier Health Sciences, Edinburgh (2019)

Jenicek, M.: A Primer on Clinical Experience in Medicine: Reasoning, Decision Making, and Communication in Health Sciences. CRC Press, Boca Raton (2012)

Mongtomery, K.: How Doctors Think: Clinical Judgment and the Practice of Medicine. Oxford University Press, Oxford (2005)

Part I
Clinical Judgment

Chapter 2
Foundations of Clinical Diagnosis

2.1 Introduction

Diagnosis is a key aspect of health care practice. The quality of diagnostic procedures has been recognized as an indicator of the quality of the entire health care system (Knottnerus et al. 2009) because appropriate diagnostics can avoid pointless treatments or mistreatments and reduce unnecessary health care costs. Thus, a critical analysis of diagnostic procedures may be both of theoretical interest and useful for empirical purposes.

Multiple disciplines are concerned with finding the best tools to establish proper diagnosis; however, the strengths and weaknesses of diagnostic procedures vary considerably across the health sciences. The term 'diagnosis' can be used to indicate either the end result of a diagnostic process, or the adopted process leading to the end result; a distinction between these two uses will be discussed in this chapter. My investigation aims to identify the underlying epistemological and ontological differences between medical diagnoses and nursing diagnoses. The structure and goals of diagnosis are elucidated in the context of clinical knowledge. The logical framework behind a diagnostic process involves identifying a condition, seeking (possible) causes of a disease (or, more generally, some negative and troublesome events), and establishing a plausible prognosis leading to an appropriate treatment. A clinical diagnosis has, of course, different goals from other types of diagnoses, even though all diagnoses share fundamental logical aspects. A critical investigation of medical diagnosis is introduced in Sect. 2.2, where it is clarified that its main purpose is to identify a biological alteration (be it organic or functional) and provide a possible helpful treatment, whereas a nursing diagnosis aims to enhance an individual's self-care, as shown in Sect. 2.3. Section 2.4 discusses the main normative facets associated to a diagnosis. Section 2.5 introduces the general notion of diagnostic framework. Its consequences in medicine are then explored in Sect. 2.6 and in nursing, Sect. 2.7.

D. Chiffi, *Clinical Reasoning: Knowledge, Uncertainty, and Values in Health Care*, Studies in Applied Philosophy, Epistemology and Rational Ethics 58, https://doi.org/10.1007/978-3-030-59094-9_2

Finally, some epistemological considerations and ontological differences between medical and nursing diagnoses are highlighted in the conclusion.

2.2 Medical Diagnosis

A diagnostic process consists of a sequence of operations with varied timing and orders that involve information-gathering and the formulation of clinical judgements. The structure of a diagnosis will depend on what time perspective it intends to adopt. In fact, it has a present-oriented focus when its purpose is to acknowledge a cluster of events associated with a disease; it is past-oriented when it attempts to isolate possible causes of a disease, and finally future-focused when it indicates a possible prognosis and an appropriate treatment for a given patient. The aim of the diagnostic process is to formulate a clinical judgment in order to:

1. identify or rule out a disease;
2. explain the findings and their likely causes to the patient;
3. predict the disease's course; and
4. modify its predicted course (Federspil and Vettor 1999).

(1) A diagnosis reflects the existing medical knowledge on a given pathological condition (Bieganski 1897). It has an evaluative dimension because the end product of the diagnostic process is a judgment (and not just a description), and judgments need to be justifiable. Ideally, the identification and thorough understanding of a disease relies in knowing the type of organic or functional alteration, its anatomopathological nature and causes, and some individual features of the patient in question (Scandellari 1991). The causes of a disease may not be known, and the available knowledge might relate only to some associations that are considered as risk factors. Be that as it may, it is only when the causes of a disease have been ascertained scientifically that the doctor can acknowledge them (Murri 1972). In this sense, *knowledge* differs from *acknowledgement*. The doctor therefore has to choose from a finite number of hypotheses to reach a clinical judgment. It seems that the doctor needs to know the causes of a disease, and not just to be able to explain a pathological condition. An explanation functionally correlates two phenomena by means of some covering laws and initial conditions (Hempel 1965), whereas in medicine causes are ascertained primarily on the strength of a codified knowledge of the pathophysiological mechanism(s) contributing to the onset of a disease, although associated social, genetic or environmental factors cannot be ruled out. When certain symptoms frequently occur together and a common but unknown cause is assumed to induce them, doctors call this condition a "syndrome".

Apart from very unlikely pathognomonic situations in which patients show a sign that is indicative of a given disease, doctors generally have to enumerate (at least partially) a finite number of possible hypotheses codified on the strength of medical knowledge, and then identify the most plausible among them, H, to test. H is thus the object of an empirical assessment that may lead to its confirmation or rejection, or—more often than not—to the production of evidential (and probabilistic) support for it. An attempt at diagnostic verification strives to produce positive and conclusive evidence of a hypothesis, also seeking evidence to support the hypothesis in other organ systems. Likewise, a diagnosis may be reached by ruling out factors that imply the presence of a disease in order to reject a given hypothesis (Langlois 2002). Either way, medical knowledge[1] is gained under a veil of uncertainty.

Doctors are not often called to create completely new diagnostic hypotheses; they need to acknowledge (at least partially), enumerate and control them. Some hypotheses can be excluded from the diagnostic process, for instance, by means of laboratory tests and somatic analyses. The collection and investigation of notable signs (usually called "anamnesis") must also be done in the light of a set of initial working hypotheses, otherwise operational errors are liable to affect the diagnostic process. Some examples of operational errors associated with the diagnostic process include those situations in which a diagnosis is unintentionally delayed (sufficient information was available earlier), is wrong (a misdiagnosis is established before the right one), or is missed (no diagnosis is made) (Graber et al. 2005). In addition to the heuristics and biases associated with probabilistic reasoning in medicine (Kahneman 2003), some diagnostic errors may relate to diagnostic uncertainty that concerns a disease's definition; measurement errors; a lack of evidence of the clinical validity of a test or of the clinical utility of a treatment; failure to consider all the diagnostic possibilities; different elicitation of experts' beliefs; and so forth (Djulbengovic et al. 2011). All these aspects prove to be misleading and affect a doctor's ability to arrive at a sound clinical judgment.

(2) In ordinary medical communications, patients and health professionals may have diverging narrative attitudes towards health problems, particularly in the time leading up to a diagnosis (Schleifer and Vannatta 2006). While the doctor's attitude is more often characterized by a scientific knowledge-based approach, the patient is oriented towards a biographical conceptualization of his or her illness. Just the same, clinical practice has also an ideographical dimension related to an individual's human and social features, and although clinical activity relies heavily on scientific outcomes and methods within a logical and probabilistic framework, it can be defined more as an art than as a science. It is quite common, in fact, for probabilities to be used when reporting a diagnosis to a patient because most diagnoses are uncertain and exposed to the risk of error. The (final) clinical probability of a diagnosis is ultimately placed in a Bayesian framework at the crossover point between the (initial) epidemiological prevalence of a disease in a population of interest and the probability of the disease given the signs observed in a given patient. Note that incidences are frequencies, while other probabilities express a degree of rational conviction, making it difficult to cope with different types of probabilities (Giaretta and Chiffi 2013). Therefore, when it comes to communicating a diagnosis to a patient, there may be some cognitive biases due to the use of different types of probabilistic information, which can easily be misunderstood.

---

[1] On the construction of medical knowledge (see Solomon 2015).

(3) A diagnosis provides goal-oriented (teleological) knowledge. Forecasting the course of a disease in a given patient is a key ingredient of clinical practice. A medical diagnosis has to provide a teleological (functional) explanation for a health-related condition. According to Nagel (1961), a function can be explained as follows: 'the function A in a system S with organization C is to enable S in environment E to engage in a process P; e.g. the heart has the function of pumping blood through the circulation system'. Alterations or losses of a health function are fundamentally important to a diagnostic judgment because a diagnosis has to (at least partially) predict the course of the patient's disease (in association with the chosen therapy) on the basis of the available evidence of the patient's health functions at the time. So, the notions of function, organization, environment and process are the key ingredients of teleological activities, and they are all time dependent. Problems in a biological system can be due to a malfunction of A, to errors in the structure of the biological system S with organization C, to negative conditions in the environment E, or to procedural errors in P. Of course, the occurrence of these conditions may be nested, and not necessarily in any given order. In a biomedical functional explanation, our main concern is to maintain the organism in equilibrium: for example, the heart's pumping action helps to keep the blood circulating and any change occurring in its circulation can deeply affect the health of the organism.

(4) The predicted course of a disease can be changed appropriately if its causes are known, and providing that it is known how to modify the disrupted function. If this is not the case, doctors have to modify a related health function that can favourably influence the situation (Bieganski 1897; Pedziwiatr 1999). In other words, many functions concur in keeping a biological system in good working order, so when doctors are unable to modify one function that is disturbed, they have to prescribe treatments designed to enhance other normal functions. From this perspective, any decision to prescribe a therapy has to be rational and focus on the patient's well-being. This can be achieved by interpreting the patient's needs on the one hand, and by grounding the diagnosis on medical knowledge within a sound logical framework on the other. Errors made within the inferential framework of a diagnosis can stem not only from the adequacy of the doctor's medical knowledge, but also from an unsound application of the laws of logic (Bieganski 1897; Pedziwiatr 1999).

The above-mentioned goals of medical diagnosis have key epistemological issues that can be elucidated by means of a rational reconstruction of the clinical diagnostic reasoning process. In the light of such pre-theoretical insights, a medical diagnosis is the prototype of any diagnostic process, in the minimal sense of the diagnosis identifying a condition, searching for its causes, forecasting its course and suggesting a treatment capable of modifying the prognosis. In the next section, I compare the medical diagnosis with a nursing diagnosis in order to show that there is an urgent need for a sound epistemological methodology also in nursing theory and practice, so as to make sense of the proprium of nursing.

2.3 Nursing Diagnosis

The nature of nursing diagnosis is an open issue. Different diagnostic systems can be found in the literature, of which the most widely used worldwide is the NANDA (North American Nursing Diagnosis Association) system, followed by its European counterpart prepared by the ICNP (International Council of Nursing Practice) and a variety of other systems based on specific nursing theories (Orem 1992; Roy and Roberts 1981; Gordon 1987). In this chapter, I will discuss the NANDA system alone. This diagnostic system is basically a taxonomy developed since 1973 for identifying and justifying nursing activities, with the purpose of adopting a standardized language for nursing diagnoses, interventions, and outcome definitions, as provided by the NNN (NANDA-NIC-NOC) association (web site: https://www.nanda.org/nanda-i-nic-noc.html). The NANDA defines a nursing diagnosis as "a clinical judgment about individual, family, or community experiences/responses to actual or potential health problems/life processes. A nursing diagnosis provides the basis for selection of nursing interventions to achieve outcomes for which the nurse has accountability" (NANDA 2012).[2] According to the NANDA, a diagnosis is closely associated with the responsibility for deciding and planning subsequent treatments. Consistent with the accepted paradigm of nursing (Fawcett and Downs 1992), and unlike a medical diagnosis, a nursing diagnosis can be community-based. For instance, the diagnosis of an "ineffective relationship" is defined as "a pattern of mutual partnership that is insufficient to provide for each other's needs". Such a diagnosis is family- or community-based, and not necessarily dependent on biological issues, which can be seen by its defining characteristics: the "inability to communicate in a satisfying manner between partners", "no demonstration of mutual support in daily activities between partners," and so forth. This has huge consequences on the nature of diagnosis in nursing. To begin with, a nursing diagnosis does not aim to isolate a specific alteration by trying to acknowledge the causes of a functional or organic alteration (as in a medical diagnosis), and does not merely rename and mimic a medical diagnosis. Nursing theory tries to integrate clinical judgment with evidence belonging to the social, psychological, philosophical and anthropological disciplines. In fact, while nursing provides a methodological interface between clinical, social and humanistic knowledge, nursing diagnoses try to address life processes taking place over time. Both medical and nursing diagnoses thus work in a tensed framework because they attempt to handle health-related processes properly in their temporal and teleological dimensions. However, a nursing diagnosis lacks certain ingredients, without which it cannot be considered a diagnosis per se:

1. a nursing diagnosis is often framed as a description of an individual's behaviour or attitude rather than as a judgment that empirically correlates causes and effects; and.

2. when a nursing diagnosis is unrelated to any biological alteration—as in the case of some forms of 'urinary incontinence', for instance—and there is no direct

---

[2]More recent versions of NANDA books do not present substantial changes.

cause/effect relationship, then it seems more like a mere empirical generalization of certain observable circumstances than a judgment based on any causal laws.

From 1 and 2, it follows that a nursing diagnosis without some form of causality (or statistical association) has no predictive power and cannot be consequently regarded as a prognostic assessment. The fact that it is not based on causal laws implies that the hypothetical reasoning used in nursing is not just a matter of choosing and confirming hypotheses. The hypothetical reasoning used in nursing frequently deals with "hypothesis-candidates" that may only be weakly supported by available evidence, precisely because of this lower reliance on casual laws.

A further weakness of the NANDA diagnostic system concerns the so-called "risk diagnoses" such as, for example, "Risk for ineffective relationship" or "Risk for spiritual distress". According to the NANDA, a risk diagnosis is "a clinical judgment about human experiences/responses to health conditions/life principles that have a high probability of developing in a vulnerable individual, family, group or community" (NANDA 2012, p. 96). If we do not wish to redefine the notions of diagnosis and risk, it is not really clear what a risk diagnosis might be. Although there are many definitions of risk, the Royal Society of London defines it as "the probability of an event together with the probability of an (uncertain) outcome, which might occur during a determined time period, in combination with the magnitude of the effect and its consequences" (Royal Society 1992). A risk diagnosis, again, does not follow the logic of an actual diagnosis because there is no acknowledgement of the individual's present conditions. There is merely a judgment on possible future events that may or may not occur, making the future prognosis depend on past causes of the condition. If the purpose of a risk diagnosis is to acknowledge a possible future condition, then it cannot—being already framed in the future—go on to predict a subsequent condition, in the sense of providing a prognosis. Following the above, a risk diagnosis would seem to be a prognosis that is used as a diagnosis without actually assessing the individual's current situation. There are also some analytical problems related to the so-called risk diagnoses and their association with the very notion of risk. Even if there is a high probability of a given event occurring (as indicated in the above-mentioned definition of risk diagnosis), this does not mean to say that the corresponding risk is necessarily high as well because the magnitude (e.g. the level of statistical association) or the consequences of such event might be negligible.

In general, the problematic aspects of nursing diagnoses relate to the difficulty of determining the prognosis which, as mentioned earlier, is inherently based on a previous diagnosis. To overcome this problem and arrive at a sound, epistemo-logically based notion of nursing prognosis, I suggest that a nursing prognosis can ideally entail choosing methods of care in order to help individuals or communities to achieve their maximal health potential, in accordance with the health status of the individual, family and community in question. By health potential I refer to individuals' capacity to provide independently for their own quality of life, given their actual state of health (Zanotti 2010; Chiffi and Zanotti 2015). I consider the notion of nurturing individuals' health potential as referring to any action to enhance their ability to control their own life processes.

Thus, nurses need interdisciplinary knowledge, logical reasoning and clinical competence to deal with the care of the whole person. Unlike its medical counterpart, a nursing diagnosis does not seem to be generated by testing a pre-set array of possible hypotheses because there is not the same reliance on causal laws. There are different ontological dimensions associated with medicine and nursing that become evident in their diagnostic judgments: respectively, the bio-functional normality in medicine, and the independence in self-care in nursing.

2.4 Diagnosis and Values

Both medical and nursing diagnoses are value-laden. Some of the normative components of the concept of diagnosis are analysed here. It is usually assumed that it is not possible to carry out a diagnosis without judgment, but the very possibility of judgment requires evaluation. What guides our diagnostic evaluations and allows us to make decisions and judgments is evidence, values and avoiding errors. Not all diagnostic errors entail negative consequences, and not all negative consequences are due to misdiagnosis, since harm may also be caused by treatment. When harm is related to misdiagnosis, then diagnostic errors may be a significant source of preventable harm (Newman-Toker and Pronovost 2009). The notion of "harm" itself also seems to be normatively laden, since the acknowledgement of a condition as harmful may depend on a system of hierarchically-organized values assigned to certain conditions. Hence, a diagnosis may encounter many normative choices before being completed. In addition, if the diagnosis is assumed to have such a normative dimension, as I believe, then it cannot be intended as a mere descriptive algorithm—either be it is conceived as a procedure or be it assumed as the final result of such a procedure—because of the value-based framework required by diagnostic reasoning.

More generally, when dealing with normativity within science, it is common to distinguish *contextual values* from *constitutive values* (Risjord 2011). Contextual values are extra-scientific even though they may influence science, whereas constitutive values are assumed to be indispensable for scientific activity. Furthermore, constitutive values can be epistemic or non-epistemic, whereby the former are commonly accepted in science, i.e. they are related to the aims of truth, knowledge, objectivity and risk reduction; and the latter are necessary to scientific work and do not present instrumental methodological validity, e.g. the concepts of wellbeing or personal development, which are non-epistemic values in the healthcare field. The existence of non-epistemic constitutive values in pure sciences may be disputed, although it is often assumed that non-epistemic normativity plays a key role in the research and practice of healthcare disciplines. It should be noted that there are cases in which an interplay exists between the epistemic and non-epistemic dimensions of normativity in science, as I will show later.

Diagnostic tests require statistical decision-making. For example, in statistical hypothesis testing, the *null* hypothesis H_0 is conventionally identified with the no-effect hypothesis to be tested. H_0 can be rejected (thus accepting in a binary context an alternative and opposite hypothesis H_1), when the *p* value (namely, the probability of obtaining a result equal or more extreme than what is actually observed assuming that H_0 is true) is equal to or less than a specified value for a statistical significance α (generally identified with a probability of 0.01 or 0.05). A type I error means that H_0 has been incorrectly rejected when H_0 is true. A type II error means that H_0 is incorrectly accepted when H_0 is false. The rate for type II error is indicated by β. In the diagnostic framework, if H_0 is the 'absence of disease' and H_1 the 'presence of disease', then type I error is a false positive diagnosis, while the type II error is a false negative diagnosis (Wulff and Gotzsche 1999).[3] Notice that the determination of the balance between thresholds for type I (false-positive) and type II (false-negative) statistical errors is an epistemic value that is called "inductive risk" (Hempel 1965) or "risk of error" (Parascandola 2010): a proper equilibrium should be achieved between statistical errors by also taking into account the sample and the effect sizes one wants to detect, e.g. a specific value of relative risk (Cranor 1990). Thus, a diagnosis is not normatively neutral even at a mere epistemological level, since it encompasses both value judgments and critical assessment of evidence. Consequently, a diagnosis may be incomplete if, for instance, the evidence is insufficient or problematic, if the evaluation is not correct according to some decision rules, if the evaluation and evidence are conflictual, etc. And although contextual values may be linked to a diagnosis, an interplay between epistemic and non-epistemic values also seems to occur in the process. Because diagnoses are constitutively probabilistic, Hempel's account of "inductive risk" (Hempel 1965)—regarding the acceptable rate of false positive and false negative results in accepting a hypothesis—may be associated with different diagnostic procedures. Imagine, for instance, the different thresholds of statistical errors (concerning the acceptable rate of false positive and false negative results) for testing a vaccine on children or on monkeys.

The interaction between epistemic and non-epistemic values is therefore possible for diagnostic and testing procedures even at a constitutive level, since the errors cannot both result lower in the same test (Cranor 1990). Hence, diagnostic procedures are normatively grounded on either epistemic or potentially non-epistemic values when they are subject to the risk of error, and this seems to hold for almost all disciplines in which decisions can be constitutively made with some risk of error. Furthermore, it is worth noting that complete, exhaustive mechanization of a diagnosis can hardly be fully achieved, since its value-based part cannot be accomplished within a mere algorithmic computation. Obviously, computational decision systems can support diagnostic decision-making to a substantial extent, even though values cannot be unconditionally confined *ex ante* to a taxonomic system of diagnostic decision-making.

---

[3]Diagnoses usually occur under a veil of uncertainty so that those who make diagnoses must develop advanced probabilistic reasoning skills given the well-known fact that intuitive probabilistic arguments are very likely to be biased (Tversky and Kahneman 1974).

A second main feature related to the concept of diagnosis is its temporal structure. A diagnosis is a sequential process explained by possible recognition of the (causal) laws governing a negative present phenomenon and by the choice of consequent possible treatments. A complete diagnostic framework that aims at reconstructing mechanisms seems to require explanations, more than just a nosographic classification of phenomena. In diagnostic frameworks, explanations are thus both causal when directed toward the past (X occurs because of Y) and teleological (also known as functional) when oriented toward the future (X occurs so that Y can occur) (von Wright 1971).

The third and last feature of a diagnosis is the teleological component associated to its explanatory power. Interestingly, it seems *prima facie* that in an etiological framework causes always precede effects, while in a teleological framework prefigured effects precede causes. Of course, a prefigured effect may not be a 'real' effect; however, it has been argued by George Henrik von Wright (1971) that teleological explanations do not seem to be always causally and temporally-based. In particular, he states that a genuine teleological behaviour in the form of "this must happen *in order* for that to occur" does not always depend on a causal relation. As von Wright (1971) pointed out:

> If, for example, I say that he ran in order to catch the train, I intimate that he thought it (under the circumstances) necessary, and maybe sufficient, to run, if he was going to reach the station before the departure of the train. This belief, however, may be mistaken – perhaps he would have missed the train no matter how fast he ran. But my explanation of his running may nevertheless be correct". (von Wright 1971, p. 84)

However, teleological explanations that are based on causality seem to provide a better justification of teleological behaviour. A different analysis of teleological behaviour is provided by Wright (1976) stating that:

> There is nothing in any of the ordinary ascriptions of goals or functions or motives or purposes or aims or drives or needs or intentions which requires us to reverse the normal cause-before-effect sequence. (Wright 1976, p. 10)

Wright's position is that teleological behaviour shows a normative and causal component, since the achievement of a goal requires the knowledge of the causes that have contributed to the occurrence of an event in the past. If the event to be reached X is caused by Y, then in order to make X happen the cause Y has to be pursued. This strategy is named '*consequence-etiology*', and is based on the idea of the demonstrated causal efficacy in the past of an event with respect to a future goal.[4] Wright (1976) clarifies that

> teleological behavior is behavior with a consequence-etiology; and behavior with a consequence-etiology is behavior that occurs because it brings about, is the type of thing that brings about, tends to bring about, is required to bring about, or is in some other way appropriate for bringing about some specific goal. (Wright 1976, pp. 37–38).

---

[4]Of course, this methodology may show some limitations in presence of deep uncertainty towards the future.

When speaking of diagnostic-related behaviours, a teleological explanation may be correct without relying in the underlying causal knowledge. For example, in diseases with unknown causes, it is possible to provide only teleological explanations. At any rate, a *complete* explanation concerning the onset of a disease can be stated when the diagnosis identifies the causes of the disease and is therefore able to restrict the options of care that provide a proper 'consequence-etiology'.

Without well-specified hypotheses, it is very difficult to undertake proper diagnostic reasoning, since the proper reason of a diagnostic judgment is to confirm or rule out a specific diagnostic hypothesis (Willis et al. 2013). Consequently, a diagnosis aims to recognise and make judgments, from signs, symptoms and other information, confirming or excluding a specific condition or disease. This has to be done by taking into account the specific goals and values of the diagnostic process.

2.5 Diagnostic Frameworks

Diagnostic soundness is extremely important because to fail in adequately considering alternative options or to have a mistaken preference for initially selected possibilities may cause considerable problems. For instance, it has been observed that an estimated 40,000 to 80,000 hospital deaths are caused by misdiagnosis annually in the US (Newman-Toker and Pronovost 2009).[5] Thus, the issue regarding the correct general structure of diagnostic reasoning and its applications has important consequences on healthcare and public health. In order to help clinicians formulate sound diagnoses, many diagnostic frameworks have been proposed.

Diagnostic frameworks are key components of many scientific and technological activities as well as of clinical practice. A diagnostic framework refers to the tools and criteria used during the diagnostic process, i.e. the equipment, set of methods or systems used to make a diagnosis. I will show how normative constraints may shape the use of normative frameworks.

When a diagnosis is considered point-like, then it may be: (a) the result of a clinical judgment or (b) the application of a diagnostic taxonomy. In case (a), the diagnosis is the final stage of a time-based process. It may be revised in the light of subsequent information, given the fallibility of any diagnosis. In case (b), since a diagnosis is merely a labelling phenomenon, it seems to be completely a-temporal. However, it can be argued that it is very unlikely that a diagnosis can be stated by an integration of the available clinical knowledge and individual expertise. There is a sort of indispensability for judgments and explanations when dealing with diagnoses. Indeed, point-like diagnoses might only be used at a high level of abstraction because what they do is to just provide categories for describing facts, and not for accurately interpreting the causal relationships among them.

---

[5]However, given the intrinsic fallibility of diagnoses and diagnostic tests, an incorrect diagnosis might be perfectly rational given the total available evidence.

I will rely on the three proposed criteria for investigating the nature of diagnostic frameworks, namely: (1) the *normative* criterion (2) the *temporal* criterion and (3) the *teleological* criterion.

Even if these three criteria might present some overlaps, I hold that they are jointly necessary for the justification of a diagnostic framework.

2.6   Diagnostic Frameworks for Medical Diagnosis

Diagnostic frameworks are analytically investigated in clinical and philosophical research and extensively used in medical practice. Errors associated with medical diagnoses are often reported in the scientific literature, giving rise to clinical, economic and social issues: for instance, it has been reported that costs related to diagnostic testing account for more than 10% of all healthcare costs (Newman-Toker et al. 2013). This also depends on the economic consequences of 'defensive medicine' malpractice, due to the recommendations for diagnostic testing which have the sole function of protecting the physician against possible negative outcomes or diagnostic errors. Indeed, ethics and soundness in the methodology of diagnostic procedures have both theoretical and empirical consequences.

In theoretical reflection of medical diagnoses, diagnoses clearly contain some normative and evaluative elements (Stempsey 1999). Engelhard (1992a) noted that "diagnoses are evaluative because concepts of disease, illness, affliction, and deformity presuppose judgments about when the minds and bodies of humans fall short of physiological or psychological ideals. To identify something as a disease or illness is to judge that it is a state of affairs that fails to realize some view of how human bodies and minds ought to be" (Engelhard 1992a, p. 75). Moreover, as already mentioned, epistemic values are associated with Hempel's inductive risk, since almost all medical diagnostic tests have a probabilistic structure. The balance between false-positive and false-negative outcomes may also be associated with extra-scientific values regarding, for instance, the choice of the proportion of cases for which it is preferable to falsely detect a disease in healthy people rather than falsely detect that there is no disease in ill people, or vice versa. Ethical problems may follow from this issue, e.g. patients and physicians may not share the same hierarchy of risks and benefits, or when choosing among different diagnoses, patients may be exposed to over-treatment or under-treatment, and so forth (Engelhardt 1992b). Differing value attributions may (at least partially) shape the clinical decisions and the interpretation of the problems, as well as outcomes and purposes in a medical diagnosis. A medical diagnosis therefore necessarily presents normative constituents, in line with the first criterion of adequacy for diagnoses, and is value-laden from an ethical point of view. Medical diagnoses are fundamental in selecting therapeutic indications, and should be used to identify and judge alterations of biological processes and of functionalities (Bieganski 1897). Bieganski, a member of the Polish school of philosophy of medicine, argued that the possibility of modifying causes of a disease is an *ideal* situation, which is not always attainable. From this perspective, diagnosis and therapy are conceived as practices, which are rational but essentially based on a scientific and logical framework (Bieganski 1897).

The second criterion of adequacy regarding the temporal structure of diagnostic frameworks is fulfilled by medical diagnostic frameworks. This may be the main reason why medical diagnoses are assumed to be the prototype of every kind of diagnosis. Still, because this type of diagnosis may be at risk of error, the physician must judge whether the diagnosis is sound enough to justify the options of care and a specific treatment (Wulff and Gotzsche 1999). Although some deviations from the main framework are possible in specific clinical contexts, the temporal component of a medical diagnosis is very well defined in the context of justification. However, notice that there are cases in which there is no attempt to explain the biological mechanism or recognise the causes of a disease in a diagnosis. Federspil (2004) calls such kinds of diagnoses "nosographic" because they only have a classificatory character within a taxonomy. That is why they can be considered as point-like rather than temporal events. Anyhow, the gold standard for medical diagnostics are the causal or "pathophysiological diagnoses" (Federspil 2004). In fact, even though some diagnoses do not explicitly refer to causality, the choice of a taxonomy and the attribution of clinical evaluations to a specific class also require some clinical judgment. Moreover, a proper classification of diseases in the health disciplines is commonly based on the explanations of biological mechanisms and causal criteria (Longo et al. 2012).

The last criterion for adequacy in diagnostic frameworks is their *teleological* function. Being value-based, the teleological objectives of diagnoses must be fulfilled. This issue is well-known in critical reflections on medical diagnostics. For instance, it has been soundly argued that "[medical] diagnosis is not knowledge for knowledge's sake. It is knowledge for the sake of action. Medicine exists in order to cure, to care, to intervene, or, in limiting cases, to know when not to intervene. Medicine is not a contemplative science" (Mainetti 1992, p. 79). Indeed, providing teleological explanations, forecasting the course of a patient's disease and administering possible treatments are the main goals of the clinical practice within medicine. This clarifies the view according to which medicine is not a speculative science but a discipline, with specific purposes and values, funded on different sciences and technologies. The ability to make a sound medical diagnosis is the most critical skill required for the exercise of this discipline, which may be grounded on diagnostic frameworks. Yet, it should be noted that diagnostic frameworks are not always successful. For instance, consider the following example of the US Preventive Services Task Force (USPSTF) recommendations for screening for breast cancer discussed in (Plutynski 2012, p. 311):

> The USPSTF recommended that women under 50 consult with their clinicians about whether to have annual screening (US Preventive Services Task Force 2009). A meta-analysis of multiple clinical trials appeared to show that the benefit for most women under 50 may be relatively small, and the cost—in terms of false positives, unnecessary biopsies, and overdiagnosis (unnecessarily treating cancers that never would have caused illness during that person's lifetime), is relatively high. For women over 50, they found that biannual screening may be as effective as annual screening for reducing age-adjusted mortality (Mandelblatt

et al. 2009; Nelson et al. 2009). As might have been predicted by more savvy publicists, the response was not positive.

According to Plutynski (2012) there are many limitations for these recommendations. The USPSTF had not sufficiently valued patients' lives or acceptable cost considerations that could influence such guidelines, violating, this way, the first criterion of adequacy for a diagnostic framework, i.e. its value-sensitiveness. Thus, risk and benefit issues that should give rise to the formulation of a diagnosis need to be refined and supplemented by some examination of the reasonable variability in values patients attach to different risks. This is particularly true when dealing with cancer, since not all cancers progress linearly or similarly. Therefore, also the second criterion of temporal adequacy is not justified. Finally, neither the third teleological criterion is fulfilled, since formulating individual clinical explanations, forecasting the course of cancer in a specific patient and administering possible treatments is not necessarily consistent with USPSTF recommendations.

2.7 Diagnostic Frameworks for Nursing Diagnosis

Expert diagnostic practice has become a growing concern for nurses, since competent diagnostic skills are assumed to be the proper basis for the later development and implementation of nursing care and decisions (Lee et al. 2006). According to some influential nursing scholars, diagnoses are often assumed to be descriptive abbreviations of clinical aspects of interest. For instance, let us analyse Marjory Gordon's perspective on nursing diagnoses, which greatly inspired the renowned NANDA system. NANDA provides a standardized language and taxonomy for nursing diagnoses, connected to interventions and outcome definitions, via the NNN organization (NANDA-NIC-NOC; website: https://www.nanda.org/nanda-i-nic-noc.html).

According to Gordon, "diagnoses are shorthand ways of referring to a cluster of signs and symptoms that occur as a clinical entity" (Gordon 1976, p. 1298). She also added that "nursing diagnoses describe health problems in which the responsibility for therapeutic decisions can be assumed by a professional nurse. In general, these problems encompass potential or actual disturbances in life processes, patterns, functions, or development, including those occurring secondary to disease" (ibidem). These definitions clearly underestimate the evaluative and normative dimension of the concept of diagnosis; that is, the first adequacy criterion. For Gordon, diagnoses are merely descriptive, and not based on judgments, values or criteria of justification. She seems to assume that a nursing diagnosis is possible if made by a nurse who has the responsibility for providing care for a specific health problem. The idea of a nurse's responsibility is mainly intended, according to Gordon, from a legal point of view (see Gordon 1987, 1998). One consequence of this assumption is that the range of possible nursing diagnoses is related to the legal (rather than the ethical) context where a nurse exercises the profession.

According to Gordon's descriptivist view, the final output of a diagnosis consists of assigning a diagnostic category (labelling) to a condition, where the diagnostic category has the following structural components: (a) the "state-of-the-patient" or "health problems"; (b) the "etiology of the problem"; and, (c) the signs and symptoms. What is missing in this view are provision for judgments and aims of diagnostic procedures. Health problems here may also be *actual* or *potential*. However, the diagnosis of a "potential problem" violates the general structure of a diagnosis, since the identification of a problem (or negative condition)—as we have seen—must actually have occurred. If the problem is placed in the future, then it raises uncertainty whether it may or may not occur. Hence, in that case, if we falsely judge something as existing in the future, then there is no sense to derive a prognosis. Diagnoses of potential problems are not genuine diagnoses, since the problem might not take place even if possible. When the concepts of prognosis and treatments are not properly taken into account in a nursing diagnostic framework (as happens in Gordon's picture), nursing diagnoses do not seem to be teleological. It is clear, in fact, that nursing knowledge must also involve an obligation to look into the future, so as to anticipate any forthcoming challenges in providing care to patients and groups (Leonard 1967). Dickoff and James (1968), for instance, firmly proposed that nursing requires teleological concepts in order to integrate nursing theory and practice. Nursing theory is a conceptual system or framework developed for some specific purposes, and is structured in levels. The lower level deals with the construction of taxonomies and causal models, while the upper one is a goal-oriented theory for nursing, called "situation-producing theory". The above authors state that "situation producing theories attempt conceptualization of desired situations as well as conceptualizing the prescriptions under which an agent or practitioner must act in order to bring about situations of the kind conceived as desirable in the conception of the goal" (Dickoff and James 1968, p. 198). Specifically, "situation-producing theory" should indicate how to create situations that match the ends of nursing (Edwards 2001). Dickoff and James also argued that, since nursing theory is oriented toward practice, it cannot be value-free; therefore, normativity cannot be dismissed in the nursing context. If normativity is a constitutive element of nursing theory, we might wonder what its constitutive values are, which still represents a very challenging issue. I will not further analyse the position of Dickoff and James, which I will thoroughly discuss in a subsequent chapter of this book; what is important to stress here is that the idea of normativity and teleological reasoning in nursing has not been properly incorporated in the frameworks guiding nursing diagnosis. Moreover, it is remarkable that "situation-producing theory" (Dickoff and James 1995) shows some similarities with Wright's (1976) 'consequence-etiology' of teleological behaviour, since both theories aim at producing or selecting those situations that are causally connected to some specific desirable aims.

Let us go back to nursing diagnoses. I have pointed out that, according to Gordon, nursing diagnosis is the mere identification of a problem in a category; this seems to be a narrow view. Gordon's perspective on nursing diagnoses does not fulfil the three necessary diagnostic criteria, meaning it can hardly support a genuine diagnosis. She considers the concept of diagnosis as one with "a useful approximation of reality"

(Gordon 1990), not as a judgment which also has a predictive aim regarding the development of a health condition based on causal laws. However, unlike medical diagnostics, it is still unclear what might count for a causal law in a nursing framework, even when one considers that "no diagnosis by itself ever made a patient better" as stated by Haynes et al. (2006, p. 277). Albeit the application of a criterion within a taxonomy may not require a judgment, a judgment regarding the internal consistency and external adequacy of a taxonomy is a prerequisite for any of its applications.

As we have already seen, a more sophisticated model for nursing diagnosis is provided by the NANDA system; the members of NANDA who worked on Gordon's ideas and definitions have then further developed such framework (NANDA 2012, p. 93).

In NANDA definitions and taxonomies, the recognition of the normative dimension as a constitutive aspect of diagnosis is still missing. The use of this taxonomy in nursing practice seems to be mostly due to the economic and insurance contributions related to nursing activity such as patient care (Doenges et al. 2010), rather than to achieve a better outcome for the patient. Critical remarks concerning the absence of any reference to values in NANDA taxonomy have been already pointed out by Lützén and Tishelman (1996). However, criticism from these two authors holds a subjectivist perspective, according to which diagnoses should be based on individualized contexts not reducible in taxonomy. In my perspective, instead, the epistemological objectivity of diagnostic frameworks is not questioned. What is also very problematic in NANDA diagnoses is that they are very often vaguely defined, hindering the same possibility of ascertaining the meanings and the causes of certain phenomena. By way of example, the NANDA diagnosis of "hopelessness" is defined as follows: "a subjective state in which an individual sees limited or no alternatives or personal choices available and is unable to mobilize energy on own behalf" (NANDA 2012–14, p. 279). The possibility of understanding the meaning and reasons why one is unable to 'mobilize energy' is at the very least vague and indefinite. One of the main factors contributing to the distinction of the reference classes in a taxonomy is *causality*. And yet, the causal laws explaining 'hopelessness' are far too vague. One might argue that NANDA diagnoses are similar to Federspil's (2004) nosographic diagnoses in medicine. Since knowledge of the causal mechanisms has a preeminent role in diagnostics, there are significant limitations in the applicability of nosographic diagnoses in the nursing domain. Nursing phenomenology is often described in ambiguous terms. For instance, the aforementioned diagnosis of "hopelessness" does not give information about the connection between causes (or statistical evidence) and observable behaviours, thus failing to appraise the usefulness of a diagnosis soundly formulated and leading to prognosis and treatment. Such a definition of 'hopelessness', in sum, does not enable the cohesion of the dynamics of causes, evidence, mechanisms and options of care. These limitations show that nursing methodology and practice need to be better grounded on a fine-grained synthesis of contents and methods from scientific, clinical and humanistic disciplines as well as by a deeper analysis of normative constraints in nursing diagnostic frameworks.

2.8   Conclusion

I have outlined the structure and goals of a diagnosis and shown that there may be some overlaps between medical and nursing judgments. I have also indicated some of the most salient elements distinguishing a nursing from a medical diagnosis.

In principle, a medical diagnosis, basically concerned with biological and functional alterations, can be established without actively involving the patient (as in emergency situations, for instance). On the other hand, a nursing diagnosis focuses on the patient's social and humanistic domains (it is context related), meaning there can be no such diagnosis without the conscious participation of the individual concerned, his/her family or the community. 'This is because the focus of nursing care is the "whole person," or persons' achievement of well-being and self-actualization' (Lunney 2012). Without a patient's participation, nursing would not be able to set achievable goals of individual development, and the nursing practice would consequently be reduced to the mere provision of supportive or substitutive care. In fact, with the patient's active involvement, it becomes possible to identify and enhance his or her own level of independence in self-care. Hence, a nursing diagnosis can give way to feasible goals for advanced nursing practices, whatever the patient's medical diagnosis may be. The practical usefulness of a diagnosis lies in providing a judgment on a patient's current situation and a prediction of potential developments in order to decide on appropriate intervention strategies.

I have critically investigated the taxonomy-based nursing diagnostic systems, which are meant to be practice oriented but lack the epistemological requirements for a proper diagnostic judgment. My analysis underscores that a nursing diagnosis should be much more than a mere descriptive algorithm to be applied uncritically. For it to enhance the quality of clinical decision making, a nursing diagnosis demands critical thinking, sound logical reasoning, and acknowledgement of the adequacy of (causal) hypotheses. I have pointed out that, although algorithmic and taxonomic decision-making tools do help support decision-making processes in the health care setting by providing well-founded scientific and clinical knowledge, they cannot replace critical thinking when diverging hypotheses or ambiguous signs exist. Still, medical and nursing diagnoses have different goals: a medical diagnosis identifies a variation from a norm, while a nursing diagnosis judges a potential mechanism for enhancing self-care.

Then, a normative stance on the structure and goals of diagnoses is presented to elucidate the constitutive aspects of diagnostic frameworks. Three essential components associated with a rational reconstruction of diagnostic frameworks were identified and critically discussed: the unavoidability of the *normative* diagnostic dimension, the *temporal* structure of the diagnostic process, and the *teleological* diagnostic perspective. On the one hand, it has been pointed out that because of the risk of statistical error in any given diagnosis, epistemic values, as Hempel's inductive risk, are always associated to diagnostics. On the other hand, within the health disciplines, non-epistemic values seem to be often adopted for diagnosis. Subsequently, a judgment-based account for diagnoses has been defended by following a rational reconstruction in my normative framework. And in order to explain the need of a teleological perspective on diagnosis and the relevance of causal laws, an analysis of Wright's (1976) notion of "consequence-etiology" has been carried out. I have shown that medical diagnoses fulfil the above-mentioned three criteria. The medical distinction between pathophysiological and nosographic diagnoses has also been discussed. In the former kinds of diagnoses the causes or the mechanisms justifying the diagnosis are explicitly stated, while in nosographic ones there is an attribution of a diagnostic class to an individual without making explicit the causal laws governing the onset and development of a disease. At any rate, I have already underlined that one of the main factors usually assumed in medical diagnostic taxonomies is the causal one.

I then examined the epistemological structure of nursing diagnoses, focusing on the perspectives of Gordon and NANDA. I described how the purpose of nursing diagnoses is directed towards individuals, families and groups, whereas that of medical diagnoses is geared towards a single patient. I have also shown that the Gordon and NANDA perspectives of nursing diagnoses do not fulfil the proposed diagnostic criteria, since there are no precise roles for constitutive values, causal laws and clinical judgments in their diagnostic frameworks. It might also be argued that these nursing diagnoses are nosographic as are the corresponding medical ones. Still, the lack of well-codified knowledge concerning the causal mechanisms that govern nursing classifications becomes a serious obstacle to the use of taxonomies for nursing diagnoses. In this sense, the possibility of grounding the teleology of nursing theory on the 'consequence-etiology' (or similar methods) is quite problematic, given the paucity of the causal accounts in the nursing diagnostic frameworks. Future research on the theory for nursing diagnosis should focus on the analysis of nursing diagnosis mechanisms, so as to connect the ontology with the epistemology of nursing theory. In conclusion, some arguments were presented to analyse the epistemological and normative foundations of nursing diagnoses in order to increase the therapeutic value of nursing knowledge.

References

Bieganski, W.: The concept of therapy. In: Löwy, I. (eds.) The Polish School of Philosophy of Medicine, pp. 91–99. Kluwer Academic Publishers, Dordrecht (1897 [1990])

Chiffi, D., Zanotti, R.: Medical and nursing diagnoses: a critical comparison. J. Eval. Clin. Pract. **21**(1), 1–6 (2015)

Cranor, C.F.: Some moral issues in risk assessment. Ethics **101**(1), 123–143 (1990)

Dickoff, J., James, P.: A theory of theories: a position paper. Nurs. Res. **17**(3), 197–203 (1968)

Dickoff, J., James, P.: A theory of theories: a position paper. Nurs. Res. **17**(3), 353–58 (1995)

Djulbegovic, B., Hozo, I., Greenland, S.: Uncertainty in clinical medicine. In: Gifford, F. (ed.) Philosophy of Medicine, vol. 16, pp. 299–356. Handbook of the Philosophy of Science. Elservier, Amsterdam (2011)

Doenges, M.E., Moorhouse, M.F., Murr, A.C.: Nursing Diagnosis Manual: Planning, Individualizing, and Documenting Client Care, 3rd edn. F.A. Davis Company, Philadelphia (2010)

Edwards, S.D.: Philosophy of Nursing. An Introduction. Palgrave, Basingstoke (2001)

Engelhardt, H.T.: The body as a field of meaning: implications for the ethics of diagnosis. In: Peset, J.L., Gracia, D. (eds.) The Ethics of Diagnosispp. 75–77. Kluwer, Dordrecht (1992a)

Engelhardt, H.T.: The emergence of the ethics of diagnoses. In: Peset, J.L., Gracia, D. (eds.) The Ethics of Diagnosis, pp. 63–71. Kluwer, Dordrecht (1992)

Fawcett, J., Downs, F.S.: The Relationship of Theory and Research, 2nd edn. Davis, Philadelphia (1992)

Federspil, G.: Logica Clinica. Mcgraw-Hill, Milan (2004)

Federspil, G., Vettor, R.: Clinical and laboratory logic. Clin. Chim. Acta **280**(1–2), 25–34 (1999)

Giaretta, P., Chiffi, D.: Causal attribution and crossing over between probabilities in clinical diagnosis. In Svennerlind, C., Almäng, J., Ingthorsson, R. (eds.) Johanssonian Investigations. Essays in Honour of Ingvar Johansson on his Seventieth Birthday, pp. 191–211. Ontos Verlag, Frankfurt (2013)

Gordon, M.: Nursing diagnoses and the diagnostic process. Am. J. Nurs. **76**(8), 1298–1300 (1976)

Gordon, M.: Nursing Diagnosis: Process and Application, 2nd edn. McGraw-Hill, New York (1987)

Gordon, M.: Toward theory-based diagnostic categories. Int. J. Nurs. Terminol. Classif. **1**(1), 5–11 (1990)

Gordon, M.: Nursing nomenclature and classification system development. Online J. Issues Nurs. **3**(2) (1998). Available: www.nursingworld.org/MainMenuCategories/ANAMarketplace/ANA Periodicals/OJIN/TableofContents/Vol31998/No2Sept1998/NomenclatureandClassification. aspx. Accessed 21.07.2020

Graber, M.L., Franklin, N., Gordon, R.: Diagnostic error in internal medicine. Arch. Intern. Med. **165**(11), 1493–1499 (2005)

Haynes, R.B., Sackett, D.L., Guyatt, G.H., Tugwell, P.: Clinical epidemiology: how to do clinical practice research, 3rd edn. Lippincott Williams and Wilkins, Philadelphia, PA (2006)

Herdman, T.H.: NANDA: International Nursing Diagnoses—Definitions and Classification (2012–2014). Wiley-Blackwell, Oxford (2012)

Hempel, C.G. (1965) Science and human values. In: Aspects of Scientific Explanation and other Essays in the Philosophy of Science, pp. 81–96. The Free Press, New York (1965)

Kahneman, D.: Maps of bounded rationality: a perspective on intuitive judgment and choice. In Frängsmyr, T. (ed.) Les Prix Nobel: The Nobel Prizes 2002, pp. 449–489. Nobel Foundation, Stockholm (2003)

Knottnerus, J.A., van Buntinx, F., Weel, C.: General introduction: evaluation of diagnostic procedures. In: Knottnerus, J.A., Buntinx, F. (eds.) The Evidence Base of Clinical Diagnosis: Theory and Methods of Diagnostic Research, 2nd edn., pp. 1–19. Blackwell Publishing Ltd., London (2009)

Langlois, J.P.: Making a diagnosis. In: Mengel, M.B., Holleman, W.L., Fields, S.A. (eds.) Fundamentals of Clinical Practice, 2nd edn, pp. 197–217. Kluwer, New York (2002)

Lee, J., Chan, A.C.M., Phillips, D.R.: Diagnostic practice in nursing: a critical review of the literature. Nurs. Health Sci. **8**, 57–65 (2006)

Leonard, R.C.: Developing research in a practice-oriented discipline. Am. J. Nurs. **67**(7), 1472–1475 (1967)

Longo, D., Fauci, A., Kasper, D., Hauser, S., Jameson, J., Loscalzo, J.: Harrison's Principles of Internal Medicine, 18th edn. McGraw-Hill, New York (2012)

Lunney, M.: Nursing assessment, clinical judgment, and nursing diagnoses: How to determine accurate diagnoses. In: Herdman, T.H. (ed.) NANDA International Nursing Diagnoses—Definitions and Classification (2012–2014), pp. 71–83. Wiley-Blackwell, Oxford (2012)

Lützén, K., Tishelman, C.: Nursing diagnosis: a critical analysis of underlying assumptions. Int. J. Nurs. Stud. **2**, 190–200 (1996)

Mainetti, J.: Embodiment, pathology, and diagnosis. In: Peset, J.L., Gracia, D. (eds.) The Ethics of Diagnosis, pp. 79–93. Kluwer, Dordrecht (1992)

Mandelblatt, J., Cronin, K.A., Bailey, S., Berry, D.A., de Koning, H.J., Draisma, G., Huang, H., et al.: Effects of mammography screening under different screening schedules: Model estimates of potential benefits and harms. Ann. Intern. Med. **151**(10), 738–747 (2009)

Murri, A.: Quattro Lezioni e Una Perizia: Il Problema del Metodo in Medicina e Biologia. Zanichelli, Bologna (1972)

Nagel, E.: The Structure of Science. Hackett, Indianapolis (1961)

Nelson, H.D., Tyne, K., Naik, A., Bougatsos, C., Chan, B.K., Humphrey, L.: Screening for breast cancer: an update for the US Preventive Services Task Force. Ann. Intern. Med. **151**(10), 727–737 (2009)

Newman-Toker, D.E: Diagnostic errors—The next frontier for patient safety. JAMA **301**(10), 1060–1062 (2009)

Newman-Toker, D.E., McDonald, K.M., Meltzer, D.O.: How much diagnostic safety can we afford, and how should we decide? A health economics. BMJ Qual Safe **22**, ii11–ii20 (2013)

Orem, D.E.: Nursing: Concepts of Practice, 3rd edn. McGraw-Hill, New York (1992)

Parascandola, M.: Epistemic risk: empirical science and the fear of being wrong. Law Probabil Risk **9**(3–4), 201–214 (2010)

Pedziwiatr, M.J.: Role of history and philosophy of medicine in the professional formation of a physician: writings of Polish School of Philosophy of Medicine. Croatian Med. J. **40**, 14–19 (1999)

Plutynski, A.: Ethical issues in cancer screening and prevention. J. Med. Philos. **37**(3), 310–323 (2012)

Risjord, M.: Nursing science. In: F. Gifford (ed.), Handbook of the Philosophy of Science. Philosophy of Medicine, vol. 16, pp. 489–522. Elsevier (2011)

Roy, C., Roberts, S.L.: Theory Construction in Nursing: An Adaptive Model. Prentice-Hall, Enflewood Cliffs (1981)

Royal Society: Risk: Analysis, Perception and Management: Report of a Royal Society Study Group. Royal Society, London (1992)

Scandellari, C.: Diagnostica. Enciclopedia Italiana (1991). Available at: https://www.treccani.it/enciclopedia/diagnostica_(Enciclopedia-Italiana)/. Last accessed 20 July 2020

Schleifer, R., Vannatta, J.: The logic of diagnosis: Peirce, literary narrative, and the history of present illness. J. Med. Philos. **31**, 363–384 (2006)

Solomon, M.: Making medical knowledge. Oxford University Press, Oxford (2015)

Stempsey, W.E.: Disease and Diagnosis: Value-dependant Realism. Kluwer, Dordrecht (1999)

Tversky, A., Kahneman, D.: Judgment under uncertainty: heuristics and biases. Science **185**(4157), 1124–1131 (1974)

von Wright, G.H.: Explanation and Understanding. Routlege & Kegan Paul, London (1971)

Willis, B.H., Beebee, H., Lasserson, D.S.: Philosophy of Science and the Diagnostic Process. Fam. Pract. **30**, 501–505 (2013)

Wrigh, L.: Teleological Explanations An Etiological Analysis of Goals and Functions. University of California Press, Berkeley (1976)

Wulff, H.R., Gotzsche, P.C.: Rational Diagnosis and Treatment: Evidence-based Clinical Decision
    Making. Blackwell Science, Malden, Ma (1999)
Zanotti, R.: Filosofia e Teoria nella Moderna Concettualità del Nursing Professionale. Piccin, Padova
    (2010)

Chapter 3
Probability in Clinical Diagnosis

3.1 Introduction

Methodologists and philosophers of medicine of Italian and Polish origin highlighted the distinction between the research activity geared towards broadening medical knowledge—possibly leading to the identification of new diseases or to the discovery of new biomedical processes—and that which is aimed at recognizing the disease or the pathological process affecting a particular individual.[1]

According to Augusto Murri (1841–1932), the accelerated progress of theoretical knowledge in medicine has contributed to a widening gap between clinical activity and pathological research. He argued that the activity of the clinician was very different from that of the pathologist. While the latter seeks to solve open problems, attempts to point up new relationships between phenomena and ends up viewing diseases as abstract entities, the former only needs to re-cognize (*riconoscere*, Italian) the disease; that is to say, to place the phenomena occurring in a patient within the context of an already codified knowledge. Murri was convinced that the clinician's task of re-cognizing might even be more challenging than that of the researcher. While the latter, in fact, can isolate a problem from contour factors, and tackle the problem with the help of an experiment, the clinician has to consider and dissect the entire set of phenomena that are present in his/her patient.

Likewise, Giovanni Federspil (1938–2010) and Cesare Scandellari (1933–) endorse Murri's distinction of the two main medical fields: pathology and clinical medicine. They also suggest that the objectives and methods of pathological research vary from those of clinical activity, although they never affirm that the biomedical knowledge of the pathologist is irrelevant to solving clinical problems.

---

[1] See Murri (1972, 2004), Antiseri (1981), Scandellari and Federspil (1985), Federspil (2004, 2010), Scandellari (2010), and Löwy (1991).

Tytus Chalubinski (1820–1889), founder of the Polish School of Philosophy of Medicine along with his colleague Edmund Biernacki (1866–1911), argued that the clinical method must be based on a holistic approach and be directed towards the care of the symptoms. According to Biernacki, in particular, the clinician's work does not require deep understanding of the phenomena that occur in the human body. He distinguishes the knowledge of the disease, which is often only partial, from its recognition. Moreover, he admits that the progress in the understanding of diseases has refined diagnostic possibilities, even if he is convinced that "knowledge about the diseases and therapeutics are independent of one another, and in fact, they exist in the doctor's mind as two different kinds of knowledge" (Biernacki 1991, p. 57). Contrary to what most doctors believe, a diagnosis is not necessary for the treatment of diseases.[2] However, Wladyslaw Bieganski (1857–1917), another member of the same Polish school, holds the opinion that the clinician cannot renounce establishing the nature of the disease affecting the patient, and that the therapeutic indications should be grounded on this judgment.

The present chapter builds upon the point of view of the aforementioned methodologists and philosophers of medicine, according to whom clinical activity has its own methods and does not intend—at least as its primary goal—to increase the knowledge of pathological science, even if it presupposes the codified knowledge of this science in order to make the correct diagnosis and then proceed to therapeutic indications.[3]

In particular, I will assume that, in certain cases, the clinician avails himself/herself of the already established causal knowledge, sometimes expressed by means of sentences of the type 'the phenomena X may be caused by Y', or 'the phenomena X are sometimes/often/always caused by Y'. I also argue, as is implicitly assumed in clinical practice, that nothing prevents in talking about the probability that the phenomena X are caused by Y. Such talk merely needs to be clarified.

The knowledge of the causes constitutes a part of the pathogenetic knowledge and certainly contributes to justifying the diagnosis. However, such knowledge is not always available. Johansson and Lynøe distinguish between the knowledge of the mechanisms "that explain how a certain event can give rise to a certain effect" (Johansson and Lynøe 2008, p. 179) and the correlation knowledge that provides "statistical associations between diseases and variables such as age, sex, profession, home environment, lifestyle, exposure to chemicals, etc." (Johansson and Lynøe 2008, p. 181). These two types of knowledge are interconnected[4]:

---

[2]Diagnostic reasoning does not occur just in medicine but also in other clinical disciplines such as nursing (see, for instance, Zanotti and Chiffi 2015) and other sciences.

[3]The Polish scholar Bieganski, who also argues for the need to provide a diagnosis and connects diagnosis and therapy, is more concerned with emphasizing the unity of medicine than with the diversity of tasks pertaining to pathology and clinical medicine.

[4]A seminal work defending the view that causal claims in the health sciences require both probabilistic dependencies and evidence for the existence of mechanisms is (Russo and Williamson 2007).

mechanism knowledge and correlation knowledge cannot only complement each other, but also interact in a way that makes both of them grow faster than they would on their own. (Johansson and Lynøe 2008, p. 182)

As suggested by Johansson and Lynøe, even correlation knowledge, when appropriately improved, can help reach a diagnostic judgment.

Whatever type of knowledge the clinician refers to, it is unavoidable for him/her to make probabilistic assessments. Additionally, it is unrealistic to expect that his/her assessments do not represent a personal opinion. It is reasonable, instead, to expect and to require the clinician to take into account the relevant statistical probabilities. When doing so, the clinician may draw inferences—called 'cross-over probabilistic inferences' by Johansson and Lynøe—in which "the premises are frequency-objective (ontological) statements and the conclusion is a subjective (epistemological) probability statement" (Johansson and Lynøe 2008, pp. 139–140). I agree entirely with this point of view, but I would also like to add that the crossover between different kinds of probabilities does not have only an inferential form. In what follows, I will provide more general analysis of this.

In clinical diagnosis, both the process of causal attribution and the crossover between probabilities may take place. I will deal with a hypothetical, yet quite realistic clinical case and will propose different idealized scenarios where the case can be applied. The possibility of causal attributions will gradually decrease, and the role of the probabilistic evaluations will change. On some of these idealized scenarios, special requirements need to be satisfied by the partition providing the point of reference for the diagnostic research. The crossover between probabilities occurs in these framings as an important, not negligible aspect.

3.2 The Clinical Case: First Version

Suppose we know that a given pathogen g rarely causes disease f. Doctors tend to express themselves in this way, without offering any overarching analysis about what it means to say that something never/rarely/ .../often/always causes something else. Let us call G the exposure to g and F the patient coming down with the disease f. As many doctors would do, we assume, moreover, that the fact that g rarely causes f implies that, with respect to the reference population, the statistical probability $P(F/G)$ is low or very low. How can one nevertheless say that, in certain specific circumstances, the event F is due to the event G? If a is the individual in question, how can one, in other words, say that in the given circumstances Fa took place[5] because of Ga? Both Fa and Ga took place, but obviously this is not enough to justify the assertion 'Fa because Ga', where the 'why' has causal meaning. May we think that in the circumstances in which the event Fa has taken place, including

---

[5] Here and in what follows I adopt this shorter way of speaking instead of referring, more correctly, to the event the sentence is about.

the previous occurrence of *Ga*, the probability of *Fa* given *Ga*, understood as a non-statistical probability, is much higher than P(F/G)? Do we thus have an example of a crossover probability?

Consider the following case. We know that the probability of a person who has eaten shellfish developing a glottal oedema is low, and we also know that James has eaten shellfish. We observe that James has developed a glottal oedema. The glottal oedema is "a pathological rare condition, allergic in nature that occurs shortly after the contact between an allergen and a sensitive subject, and admits only a few possible causes among which there is certainly the ingestion of shellfish" (Federspil 2005, p. 76).[6] Knowing that in the few hours before the onset of the glottal oedema James had not come into contact with other substances possibly containing allergens, a clinician would conclude that, with high probability, James developed an oedema of the glottis due to the ingestion of shellfish.

From the logical point of view, the clinician makes an inference based on premises, which he recognizes as true, and the inference leads him/her to recognize the truth of the conclusion that is inferred. What are the premises of the inference? If we include among them the general relevant knowledge concerning the glottal oedema, we have:

(A)   The probability that a person who has eaten shellfish shortly afterwards will develop a glottal oedema is low.
(B)   James has eaten shellfish.
(B_1)   James has a glottal oedema.
(B_2)   The glottal oedema has an allergic cause.
(B_3)   After the ingestion of shellfish, and before the onset of the glottal oedema, James did not come into contact with known allergens other than those contained in shellfish and a possible previous contact with a known allergen could not have caused the oedema.
(B_4)   The glottal oedema appeared shortly after the ingestion of shellfish.

The conclusion that is considered as being very likely is the following:

(C)   The cause of James' glottal oedema was the ingestion of shellfish.

The conclusion (C) actually appears very likely, despite the premise (A). Consequently, one might have the impression that an event, i.e. James' glottal oedema, which according to (A) is unlikely given the ingestion of shellfish, appears certainly, or almost certainly to be caused by the ingestion of shellfish. Suppose that (A) is asserted on the base of a statistical investigation. Do we have a transition from a low statistical probability to a high probability of another kind?

We cannot give an accurate response without first observing that the ingestion of shellfish, which is given in (A) as the condition of a conditional probability, is alleged

---

[6]"Glottal oedema", better known nowadays as "laryngeal oedema", is an "abnormal accumulation of fluid in tissues of any part of the larynx, commonly associated with laryngeal injuries and allergic reactions" (MeSH (Medical Subject Headings) 2018).

as something that happened to James, and is after integrated with other information, including a specific example of the type of conditioned event, i.e. James' glottal oedema. If we keep on talking in terms of conditional probability, we might be tempted to say that the supposed statistical probability $P(F/G)$ has given way to the probability of Fa given Ga and other information. There seems to be a transition from a statistical probability into a different kind of probability, though it should be noted that the transition is made while changing the content of the conditional probability.

The probabilistic analysis of the inference should be carried out in detail, but before doing so, it is worth pointing out that this type of analysis could be avoided, or brought about in a special way, if, after all the assumptions are made explicit, the inference ends up having a deductive nature.

Suppose it is considered obvious that

(C$_1$) The absence of contact with allergens other than those contained in shellfish necessarily implies that none of them can have caused James' oedema.

Therefore, the falsity of the conclusion (C) is only possible, despite the truth of the premises (B)–(B$_4$), if one admits to the possibility that James' oedema depends on an allergen, which is unknown to us but which he came into contact with. In fact, from (B$_1$) and (B$_2$) it follows that the oedema of the glottis is only due to the action of an allergen; (B$_3$) states that shellfish contain the only known allergens James had contact with and which could have caused the oedema; and (B$_4$) states that the time between the ingestion of shellfish and the appearance of the glottal oedema was short, thus seeming to exclude—with high probability but still in a way that is difficult to determine—that James could have come into contact with an unknown allergen such as to cause the oedema of his glottis. If this possibility is ruled out, (A) does not seem to have any role in the justification of (C); thus, we can share Federspil's statement that "the conclusion is not based on the probability inherent in the law invoked" (Federspil 2005, p. 76).[7] Assuming that

(C$_2$) James did not come into contact with any unknown allergen,

we can point out that the piece of reasoning that was implicitly carried out appears to be deductive in nature.[8]

Of course, being able to reach a diagnostic conclusion by deductive inference does not guarantee the certainty of the conclusion. The conclusion of a deductive inference is certain if all of its premises are certain. Since this is not always the case, then neither can the conclusion gained through deductive reasoning always be certain. The case of premises not all being certain is quite common, but we cannot always

---

[7] There is a clear similarity between the case described by Federspil and the famous case of paresis due to syphilis adduced by Scriven (1959) in order to show that the causal attribution does not presuppose the high predictability of the caused effect.

[8] Note that (C$_2$) can be suggested, of course not justified, by (B$_4$), and that it bereaves (B$_4$) of any role from the deductive point of view.

notice the non-certainty of a premise. For example, it may be difficult to notice it in the deductive inference from (B)–(B$_3$) and (C$_1$)–(C$_2$) to (C). Consider, in particular, the premises (B$_2$), (B$_3$) and (C$_2$). (B$_2$) is a general statement concerning the cases of glottal oedema. Unless the definition of a glottal oedema assumes that its only possible causes are allergens, it cannot be excluded that there might be cases of this disease that do not have an allergic cause. Concerning (B$_3$), its reliability depends, among other things, on an investigation based on indirect observations, which were not made by the clinician but reported to him, and which might be insufficient to exclude contact with other known allergens. (C$_2$) appears to be plausible, given the breadth of available knowledge about the possible allergens, but it obviously cannot be accounted for as certain.

If the uncertainty of a sentence s is defined as 1-prob(s), where 'prob' is an appropriate notion of the probability for sentences, we know that the uncertainty of a deductive conclusion does not exceed the total uncertainty of the premises, given by the sum of the uncertainties of the individual premises. In short, the uncertainty does not increase when validly inferring the conclusion. It can remain the same if the premises are consistent and if all of them are essential for the validity of the deductive conclusion (Adams 1975, 1998; Hájek 2001). Consequently, in general, a deductive conclusion is less uncertain the less uncertain its premises are. It follows that assumptions that are more or less plausible (though not certain), and that are too often taken for granted, may attribute to the conclusion a degree of uncertainty that is too high compared to what is reasonably required for a clinical diagnosis and a choice of therapy.

However, is it adequate to define the uncertainty of a sentence s as 1-prob(s)? For the sake of argument, let us assume that it is, even if in the case under analysis, the probability concerns (also) sentences stating relations of causation, which is knowingly a complex and controversial issue. We agree that it is not clearly evident how to find a way to assign a probabilistic value to a statement of causation such as (C). An objective sense can be suggested by the fact that an allergen acts only under certain conditions, so that one might think to look for the percentage of the cases where such conditions are satisfied among the cases of contact with the allergen. On the other hand, the fact that these conditions are generally not known, or cannot be ascertained, seems to give room for the application of a subjective-epistemic notion of probability.

At any rate, it has to be kept in mind that clinicians have to express themselves about particular cases on the basis of what they believe, and what they believe depends on their expertise and scientific background. Thus, it seems only natural to interpret the probabilistic assessments of the clinician about a particular case in an epistemic-subjective sense, as confidence levels based on personal opinions and knowledge. This calls the question of how the clinician should be influenced by the available 'objective' scientific and statistical knowledge. It is a difficult and complex problem, which I will try to deal with in the next sections.

3.3 The Clinical Case: Second Version

Suppose that the clinician does not have any doubt about the allergic nature of the glottal oedema, hence he/she accepts (B_2), but he/she is not willing to hold (B_3) (after the ingestion of shellfish, and before the onset of the glottal oedema, James did not come into contact with known allergens other than those contained in shellfish, and a possible previous contact with a known allergen could not have caused the oedema) because he/she is not sure of the reliability of the investigation that was carried out to establish (B_3). The clinician might even doubt that the particular piece of shellfish eaten by James contained any allergens. The deduction of (C) is no longer possible, thus the possibility of evaluating the probability of (C) based on how the uncertainty of the premises is transmitted to the conclusion through deductions, is no longer available.

Can the clinician calculate the probability of (C) in a different way? Let us observe at the outset that the problem is not to determine how high the conditional probability is that James will have an oedema of the glottis given that he has ingested shellfish. When identified with the statistical probability of a glottal oedema given the ingestion of shellfish, this probability is low and, in any case, cannot in itself adequately represent a relation of causation. On the other hand, if it is assumed—from a Bayesian point of view—that both James' glottal oedema and his previous ingestion of shellfish are acquired as entirely certain information, then the probability of each one of the two events is to be updated to 1 and, therefore, even the conditional probability of the former event given the latter is to be updated to 1.

One might even decide to disregard any understanding of the relation of causation and may simply say that the statement (C) is justified to the extent that the oedema event is predictable from the ingestion of shellfish, according to the classical approach of the 'received view' in philosophy of science. Yet, if we only rely on the statistical probability of the glottal oedema given the ingestion of shellfish, the absence of an oedema, rather than its appearance, is also predictable. Additionally, the absence of an oedema would have been predictable with even higher probability, if one were able to verify with certainty that James did not come into contact with any other (known or unknown) allergen. Perhaps the knowledge of certain physiological features of James would have allowed the clinician to make a reliable prediction of the appearance of the glottal oedema, but such knowledge was not (and is not) available.

I assume that the relation of causation cannot be eliminated or reduced to other notions, and I will consider how it is possible to assign a probabilistic value to the causal statement (C). Note that the clinician already knows that James has a glottal oedema. His/her final objective is not to ascertain the degree of probability for James to develop the oedema after the ingestion of shellfish, but rather to treat the oedema; in this sense it may be useful for the clinician to know what has caused the oedema in order to remove it. The etiological knowledge may also be useful for preventing future oedemas, which could represent an additional motivation for the search of the cause.

Since the clinician cannot ascertain the cause with complete certainty, he/she can try to ascertain what the probabilities of the single possible alternative known causes are; that is, for each possible cause, the clinician can assess the conditional probability of the oedema given the cause and the other relevant information. Based on such probabilities, the clinician can easily see which one holds the highest rank.

In this situation, the clinician is faced with two problems. In the first place, the conditional statistical probability of a possible cause, given the morbid phenomenon, is not often immediately available. Secondly, the clinician must take into account what he/she knows about James. Regarding the first issue, the inverse probabilities of the morbid phenomenon given the possible cause and the initial epidemiologically based probabilities can be more readily known. Suppose that these probabilities are known, and therefore the requested conditional probabilities may be indirectly reconstructed from them. In order to consider the special features of James—this is the other problem to deal with—the clinician could transform these probabilities into subjective-epistemic probabilities. By benefitting from a basic idea by Salmon and applying Bayesianism, the clinician may proceed as follows.

I refer to as large as possible a population R of individuals who came into contact with at least one known allergen, and I call A the property of having a glottal oedema. For each set of known allergens, consider the property of having come into contact with the allergens of the set. For the sake of simplicity, I assume that there are only two allergens, c_1 and c_2, corresponding to the C_1 property of having been in contact with c_1 and the C_2 property of having been in contact with c_2. The properties to be considered are therefore $C_1 \wedge \neg C_2$, $C_2 \wedge \neg C_1$ and $C_1 \wedge C_2$. Call, respectively, K_1, K_2 and K_3, their restrictions to R^9 and suppose that the statistical probabilities $P(A/R)$ and $P(A/K_i)$, $1 \leq i \leq 3$, are known. Suppose also that $P(A/K_i) \neq P(A/R)$ for all i. It follows that every property K_i is *statistically relevant* for A within R, following Salmon's definition of this notion. According to the way in which K_i has been introduced, and based on the shared scientific knowledge, K_i (with $i \leq 3$) can have causal efficacy for A; namely, having the property K_i may causally determine having the property A, since c_1 or c_2 can cause the oedema of the glottis. Even if K_3 is defined by the exposure $C_1 \wedge C_2$, the causal role of K_3 may be due to the causal efficacy of only c_1, of only c_2 or of both c_1 and c_2. Assume that for the cases of oedema in K_3 it is not possible to identify which of these possibilities took place.

Let us wonder whether, based on the already acquired knowledge—that is, the scientific knowledge s and evidence e—we know some conditions F contributing to the causation of the glottal oedema, such that $P(A/K_i \wedge F) > P(A/K_i)$. If the answer is negative, we say that the class described by K_i is epistemically and causally homogeneous with respect to A, s and e. If, for each i, the class described by K_i is epistemically and causally homogeneous with respect to A, s and e, the partition K of R in K_1, K_2 and K_3 is epistemically and causally homogeneous with respect to A, s and e.

The main distinction between the notion of homogeneity and that of Salmon regards the restriction of the quantification to the conditions that have a causal role

---

[9] A, K_1, K_2 and K_3 isolate certain classes to which I refer in the same manner.

for the *explanandum*. Of course, speaking of a causal role introduces some lack of clarity that the context may eliminate partially, but not completely. On the other hand, there now seems to be a broad consensus that it is not possible to provide an eliminative reduction of the relation of causation. In addition, because of the irreflexivity of the causation relation, speaking of a condition F endowed with causal role for the *explanandum* A is advantageous for immediately excluding that A itself may be regarded as one of the conditions F by which to assess the homogeneity of the classes of the considered partition.

Is the concept of epistemic causal homogeneity useful to the clinician dealing with James' case? K_i is epistemically and causally homogeneous with respect to A, if any further causal specification of K_i is not known such as to make A more likely. The idea that we want to capture is that having the property K_i is known as causally contributing to having A, and there is nothing more that one can know about it.

If James has the property K_i, if K_i is epistemically and causally homogeneous with respect to A, and if that is known as a part of the total available evidence, it is reasonable to require that the clinician assigns to James a probability of developing a glottal oedema that depends on the statistical probability $P(A/K_i)$. More precisely, if James is called j, it is natural to require and to assume that the subjective probability p of the clinician and the evidence e available to him/her are such that:

(i) $p(Aj/e) = p(Aj/(K_ij \wedge P(A/K_i) = q))$

that is, the subjective probability that the clinician assigns to Aj given e is determined by the subjective probability of Aj given both K_ij and $P(A/K_i) = q$, where $P(A/K_i)$ is the statistical probability of A in K_i.[10] If it is certain that $P(A/K_i) = q$, then $p(Aj/(K_ij \wedge P(A/K_i) = q)) = p(Aj/K_ij)$. Moreover, we assume that no other relevant information is available, so that it is also natural to assume:

(ii) $p(Aj/K_ij) = q$

that is, the subjective probability of Aj given K_ij has the same value q as the statistical probability $P(A/K_i)$.[11]

If we already know that James had a glottal oedema and that he belongs moreover to a specific K_i, then the knowledge of the causal role of K_i justifies a corresponding attribution of causality, even when $P(A/K_i)$ is low.[12] In this case, the value of the statistical probability $P(A/K_i)$ does not have any significant role, as it falls within the deductive reconstruction of the argument.

However, we are now considering the case in which the clinician does not accept (B3) and therefore does not know that James belongs to a specific subclass K_i. For

---

[10] I am assuming the possibility of a fully subjective interpretation of probability, including conditional probability and a posteriori probability.

[11] See (Festa 2004, p. 60 and p. 64). I emphasize the assumption that the statistical probabilities have been correctly determined and are certain.

[12] More precisely: James's assignment to K_1 justifies the identification of the cause of his oedema with c_1, James' assignment to K_2 justifies the identification of the cause of his oedema with c_2, James' assignment to K_3 leaves open any causal attribution.

each subclass K_i, the clinician may have uncertain evidence of James' belonging to K_i. Suppose, for example, that his/her subjective evaluations are the following:

$$p(K_1j) = 0.4$$
$$p(K_2j) = 0.5$$
$$p(K_3j) = 0.1$$

In general, the subjective evaluations of the clinician can vary within a very wide range, but they should be compatible with a correct use of the available information. Notably, the clinician should not assess James' belonging to a specific K_i as being more likely only because (using the example) the oedema of the glottis would be statistically more likely in K_i. The incorrectness of such an assessment should be intuitively evident if we consider the case of a K_i with very few elements. The possible higher level of probability of A in K_i can surely not be a reason for considering James' belonging to K_i as more likely.

Concerning the conditional probabilities of the type $p(Aj/K_ij)$, let us continue to assume that the total evidence available to the clinician is not such as to make $p(Aj/K_ij)$ different from $P(A/K_i)$. For purely illustrative purposes, we can suppose that the clinician endorses the following, completely hypothetical, conditional probabilities:

$$p(Aj/K_1j) = 0.2$$
$$p(Aj/K_2j) = 0.1$$
$$p(Aj/K_3j) = 0.3$$

From Bayes' theorem, it follows that:

$$p(K_1j/Aj) = (0.4 \times 0.2)/(0.4 \times 0.2 + 0.5 \times 0.1 + 0.1 \times 0.3)$$
$$= 0.08/(0.08 + 0.05 + 0.03) = 0.08/0.16 = 0.5$$
$$p(K_2j/Aj) = (0.5 \times 0.1)/0.16 = 0.05/0.16 = 0.31$$
$$p(K_3j/Aj) = (0.1 \times 0.3)/0.16 = 0.03/0.16 = 0.18$$

Thus, the probability of belonging to the class K_1 given the glottal oedema is greater than the other conditional probabilities of the same type. Since there is a causal significance of K_1 with respect to A, it seems reasonable to conclude that the probability that C_1 caused James' oedema is the highest because the probability of James' belonging to K_1 (given his oedema) is the highest.

3.4   The Clinical Case: Third Version

Suppose now that the initial uncertainty is even greater. The clinician does not accept (B_3) (after the ingestion of shellfish and before the onset of the oedema of the glottis,

James did not come into contact with known allergens other than those contained in shellfish, and previous contact with a known allergen could not have caused the oedema). The clinician does not even accept (C_2) (James did not come into contact with any unknown allergens), as he/she is not willing to exclude any unknown-allergen contact for James. Obviously, the deduction of (C) is not possible and, again, it is no longer possible to assess the probability of (C) based on the way in which the uncertainty of the premises is transmitted to the conclusion through deductions.

The (partial) statistical-causal analysis proposed above cannot be reapplied without incurring in major changes.

In this case too, we assume that the known allergens are only c_1 and c_2, corresponding to the property C_1 of having been in contact with c_1 and to the property C_2 of having been in contact with c_2. The reference class is a population R, which this time includes individuals who have not come into contact with any known allergen. Thus, four properties need to be considered: $C_1 \wedge \neg C_2$, $C_2 \wedge \neg C_1$, $C_1 \wedge C_2$ and $\neg C_1 \wedge \neg C_2$. For each of their restrictions to R—call them, respectively, K_1, K_2, K_3 and K_4—let us suppose that we know the statistical probability $P(A/K_i)$, $1 \leq i \leq 4$, given by the frequency of A in K_i. If $P(A/K_i) \neq P(A/R)$, the property K_i is statistically relevant for A within R.

Assume that for each $i \leq 3$ $P(A/K_i) > P(A/R)$, but $P(A/K_4) < P(A/R)$. K_1, K_2 and K_3 may have causal efficacy for A in the same sense that is assumed above. However, it is difficult to argue that K_4, namely $\neg C_1 \wedge \neg C_2$, has causal efficacy for A. The clinician is convinced that A may also have causes other than c_1 or c_2, but he/she is oblivious to how many or what they may be. In addition, since $P(A/K_4) < P(A/R)$, K_4 does not make A more likely.

Suppose, for each $i \leq 4$, and therefore also for $i = 4$, that no conditions F are known, which are endowed with causal efficacy for A and are such that $P(A/K_i \wedge F) > P(A/K_i)$. Still, since it is not possible to provide any reason for the causal role of K_4, K_4 cannot be regarded as epistemically and causally homogeneous with respect to A and to the available knowledge. Then, it is not even possible to consider the partition K of R in K_1, K_2, K_3 and K_4 as epistemically and causally homogeneous with respect to A and to the available knowledge.

It may, therefore, not be possible to assign a higher probability to a specific causal attribution. This takes place when James comes out as most likely belonging to the class K_4. Suppose, for example:

$$p(K_1 j) = 0.1 \quad p(Aj/K_1 j) = 0.4$$

$$p(K_2 j) = 0.2 \quad p(Aj/K_2 j) = 0.5$$

$$p(K_3 j) = 0.1 \quad p(Aj/K_3 j) = 0.6$$

$$p(K_4 j) = 0.6 \quad p(Aj/K_4 j) = 0.2$$

It follows that:

$$p(K_1j/Aj) = (0.1 \times 0.4)/(0.1 \times 0.4 + 0.2 \times 0.5 + 0.1 \times 0.6 + 0.6 \times 0.2)$$
$$= 0.04/(0.04 + 0.1 + 0.06 + 0.12) = 0.04/0.32 = 0.12$$
$$p(K_2j/Aj) = (0.2 \times 0.5)/0.32 = 0.1/0.32 = 0.31$$
$$p(K_3j/Aj) = (0.1 \times 0.6)/0.32 = 0.06/0.32 = 0.18$$
$$p(K_4j/Aj) = (0.6 \times .2)/0.32 = 0.12/0.32 = 0.37$$

In this case, James' probability of not having come into contact with any of the known allergens is the highest. Note moreover that upon admission of the existence of an unknown allergen, even the certainty of contact with the known allergen does not rule out another possible contact with an unknown allergen, and that the latter may have caused the oeadema.

3.5   The Clinical Case: Fourth Version

How should one proceed when one observes a glottal oedema in the case—entirely fictional—in which no possible cause is known? Suppose that the clinician knows only that certain conditions favour the appearance of the oedema; namely, that the oedema is more frequent among those who satisfy at least one of certain conditions. In epidemiological terms, we can say that we only know of some risk factors for the oedema of the glottis. In general, risk factors cannot be considered as causes and their knowledge might have no utility in terms of diagnosis and treatment. Suppose, however, that certain conditions are useful in determining the type of oedema, the prognosis and possibly the treatment. In this case, it is natural to try to determine the condition that favoured James' oedema, as it would be useful information from a clinical point of view, even if it would not suffice to identify a cause with certainty and precision.

But what type of conditions are we to consider? The clinician should draw information from his/her pathological and epidemiological knowledge, while being guided by some methodological principles that are justified by general epistemological considerations. In particular, although in the case imagined it is not possible to speak of causes, but only of favourable conditions, it is natural to rule out those conditions that do not satisfy some formal properties of the causes, even if the conditions that were not excluded cannot be qualified as causes. In particular, D can be a cause of E neither if it takes place after E, nor if both D and E are direct effects of a third event C (a conjunctive fork).

In continuation, we will only touch upon some basic ideas proposed by Hans Reichenbach and Patrick Suppes, with the understanding that the line of research they set forth does not necessarily lead to a satisfactory notion of probabilistic causality. The main concerns in Reichenbach's and Suppes' proposals are distinguishing between correlations and causality, and recovering an asymmetrical probabilistic causal relation so as to have the probabilistic cause preceding the probabilistic effect.

The first problem concerns the conjunctive fork, which is defined by Reichenbach as follows:

1. $0 < P(C) < 1$.
2. $P(D \wedge E/C) = P(D/C) P(E/C)$.
3. $P(D \wedge E/\neg C) = P(D/\neg C) P(E/\neg C)$.
4. $P(D/C) > P(D/\neg C)$.
5. $P(E/C) > P(E/\neg C)$.

Condition 1 states that the probability of the event C is in the open interval $(0,1)$, conditions 2 and 3 state that D and E are probabilistically independent with respect to C and to $\neg C$, while conditions 4 and 5 state that C is positively relevant for both D and E. It is often said that C and $\neg C$ screen off D from E. Conditions 1–5 entail 6:

6. $P(D \wedge E) > P(D)P(E)$; namely, there is a positive correlation between D and E, but this is due to the common 'cause' C.

Thus, if there is a positive correlation between D and E and there is an event C which satisfies 1–5, then C is a (probabilistic) cause for both D and E; and this fact explains the lack of independency between D and E (Reichenbach 1956).[13]

Regarding the second problem, Suppes assumes, as a primitive fact, that a cause temporally precedes its effects. On this basis, he introduces the idea of a *prima facie* 'cause' such that when it occurs, it increases the probability of the effects (Suppes 1970). Suppes states that C at t', shortly $C_{t'}$, is a *prima facie* 'cause' of E at t, shortly E_t, if and only if:

$t' < t$
$P(C_{t'}) > 0$
$P(E_t/C_{t'}) > P(E_t)$, which holds only in cases where $P(E_t/C_{t'}) > (E_t/\neg C_{t'})$ holds.

He later defines a strong notion of a spurious cause as follows: $C_{t'}$ is a spurious 'cause' of the event E_t if and only if $C_{t'}$ is a *prima facie* 'cause' of E_t and there is a partition $\{K_{1,t''}, K_{2,t''}, ..., K_{n,t''}\}$ such that
$t'' < t'$

---

[13]It has been observed that, when more events screen off D from E, the notion of the conjunctive fork is not sufficient to individuate a common cause (Uffink 1999); but I will not go into this issue herein.

$P(E_t/C_{t'} \wedge K_{i,t''}) = P(E_t/K_{i,t''})$, where i is a natural number belonging to [1, n].

A genuine cause is a non-spurious *prima facie* 'cause'.

The search for a satisfactory notion of probabilistic causality[14] continued; plus, attempts were made to face the many paradoxes that were more or less associated with it (the Simpson Paradox, the Lindrey–Jeffrey Paradox, etc.). In the following, we hint at a simple way in which the basic idea of screening off –already tacitly applied—might be slightly modified by adding a temporal reference, and may then be used for diagnostic purposes in the new imaginary version of our case, where no proper causal knowledge is assumed to be available.

The reference class is made up of a population R, which we assume to be divided on the basis of the conditions C_1 and C_2 in such a way that the properties $C_1 \wedge \neg C_2$, $C_2 \wedge \neg C_1$, $C_1 \wedge C_2$ and $\neg C_1 \wedge \neg C_2$ determine a partition K in the corresponding classes K_1, K_2, K_3 and K_4. Let $K_{i,t}$ be the class of the instances of K_i at t and $A_{t'}$ the class of instances of A at t', where $t < t'$. We can request that $K_{i,t}$ should be considered as a condition that favours $A_{t'}$ only if[15] there is no known condition C_{t*}, defined on R, where $t* < t$, such that C_{t*} screens off $K_{i,t}$ from $A_{t'}$. Then, the diagnostic process may proceed as above, transforming statistical probabilities of the form $P(/)$ into a subjective-epistemic probability of the form $p(/)$ with the aim of seeking for which $K_{i,t}$ $p(K_{i,t}j/A_{t'}j)$ is the highest.

Note that also other requirements, formulated to reach a satisfactory concept of probabilistic causality, can or should help lead the search towards an informative condition about the pathology affecting a patient (when its origin and evolution are widely unknown).

3.6   A Final, Though not Minor Problem

The classes into which the reference population has been partitioned correspond to the number of hypotheses about the cause or condition that have favoured James' oedema. The assignment of James into any of these classes has an initial plausibility that the clinician can quantify by means of probabilistic values representing the extent of his/her initial confidence in their truth. As emphasized above, these values should be used as the basis by which to calculate the probability of James' belonging to each class, given the oedema.

As stated by Johansson and Lynøe, "it is difficult, not to say impossible, to ascribe numerical values to epistemic statements" (Johansson and Lynøe 2008, p. 134). However, there are procedures that may help the clinician explicitly and soundly to assess the epistemic initial probabilities.

---

[14]The original motivation for this line of research was a reductionist one. See (Salmon 1980) for a critique of such motivation, which is now generally abandoned.

[15]What follows 'only if' is proposed as a necessary condition that is open to further specification.

Note that it is also possible that the clinician's assessment of the initial probability ends up being inconsistent. The so-called expert elicitation can be applied to single out and eliminate potential inconsistencies. Many techniques of eliciting probabilities are available (Slottje et al. 2008): according to one of these, the expert is asked to evaluate whether the actual value of a quantity is higher or lower than a certain number. This can be carried out, for instance, by means of graphical tools such as probabilistic wheels. Alternatively, the expert is asked to fix the value of a quantity such that the probability of higher or lower values turns out to be some specific amount. We will not go into the analysis of these techniques; what is important for the present discussion is that the clinician be aware of the possibility of coming across inconsistencies and also of the availability of some methods for avoiding them.[16]

Moreover, even if clinician's assessments of the probabilities relevant to a specific clinical problem comply with the rules of probability calculus, they might nonetheless turn out to be arbitrary, at least to a certain extent. Arbitrariness should be limited, and in fact it can be reduced by taking into account the epidemiological information. Of course, epidemiological data is not always *relevant* when dealing with a clinical case. It seems reasonable to hold that it may be relevant for the analysis of a clinical case when some of the following conditions are fulfilled (Lagiou et al. 2005):

1. The exposure to risk factors is also an established cause of the disease;
2. The exposure of the individual is similar (as regarding duration, intensity, latency) to the exposure causing the disease;
3. The disease of the individual must be similar to that which is etiologically associated with the exposure;
4. The individual has not to be exposed to other risk factors; and.
5. The relative risk (RR)—namely, the ratio of the probability of the disease in the exposed population to that in the unexposed population—must be greater than 2. If the RR is lower than 2, then the association between the exposure to the risk factor and the disease needs to be carefully analysed and methodologically motivated, since a weak association does not rule out the possibility of the clinical relevance of such an association.

These conditions must not be seen as robust criteria supporting the use of epidemiological data in the clinical context, but rather as constraints functioning as standards that guide the integration of epidemological evidence in clinical practice. It is important to stress that the clinician's decision-making process can greatly benefit from clinical guidelines. Of course, the clinician can break away from these guidelines if there is a reasonable motivation for a different judgment. Nevertheless, such subjective judgment, even when it is formally consistent, cannot be arbitrary but should be methodologically constrained and explicitly justifiable based on the theoretical and empirical knowledge available given the specific situation.

---

[16]However, I do not rule out the possibility that the clinician faces some kind of fundamental uncertainty in which probabilities are not well definable or computable and some forms of abductive reasoning are required (Chiffi and Pietarinen 2017).

3.7 Concluding Remarks

I discussed the role of causality and probability assignments in relation to a clinical case that seemed to be quite significant. The analysis that has been carried out is grounded on some theses about the nature of the physician's diagnostic activity. Initially, I endorsed the idea that clinical diagnosis is based on pathological knowledge that has already been acquired; clinical diagnosis in this case is not intended to extend the acquired knowledge, although it might unintentionally lead to the acquisition of information that is useful for its extension. Secondly, I observed that presupposed knowledge can be both causal knowledge and correlation knowledge. The former, in particular, concerns events that trigger disease processes and the very mechanisms by which these processes evolve. Based on classical and recent research concerning the notion of cause, I hold that this concept is not completely reducible to other concepts, and that a primitive idea of causal relationship may tacitly underlie the research of correlations that are relevant for medical knowledge.

I emphasized that the role of probability is crucial. What's more, it is crucial to assess the confidence allotted to conclusions obtained deductively from not entirely certain premises. We are bound to assume that the clinician's assignment of probability to a specific case is the result of his/her own evaluation, leading us to conclude that probabilities are to be regarded as subjective. However, it is quite natural to request nonarbitrary and (as far as possible) statistically-based probabilities.

It seems to us that in clinical diagnosis initial probabilities are more difficult to connect with statistical data. That is not surprising and, to a certain extent, is as it should be. There is, however, a problem in assuring the consistency and limiting the arbitrariness of the clinician's evaluations. I hinted at some indications, taken from the literature, which might be useful for this purpose. Some conditional probabilities are rather more easily identifiable with suitable statistical frequencies. The identification requires a high degree of normative idealization; and I derived from the literature some indications about the ideal way in which this identification can be pursued. In a less idealized approach, there might be other more general, justified ways in which the clinician may transform the conditional statistical probabilities into subjective conditional probabilities regarding the patient he/she is taking care of.

After all, it appears that two kinds of probability have a definite role: the frequency-objective and the epistemic/subjective. Is there any role for some other kinds of probability, in particular for a notion of probability as propensity or for a Baconian perspective on probability (Jonsen and Toulmin 1988; Weinstock et al. 2013) and induction? Surely, the clinician may base his probabilistic assessment of a patient having a certain disease on a more or less justified attribution of certain propensities to him/her. But is this enough, or are other reasons also needed to identify a role for a specific kind of a propensity-based singular-objective probability? I do not exclude that a deep understanding of medicine in general, not only of clinical activity, might require some room for a propensity interpretation of probability. However, a further separate and dedicated analysis would be needed.

References

Adams, E.W.: The Logic of Conditionals: An Application of Probability to Deductive Logic. D. Reidel, Dordrecht (1975)

Adams, E.W.: A Primer of Probability Logic. CSLI publications, Stanford (1998)

Antiseri, D.: Teoria unificata del metodo. Liviana, Padova (1981)

Biernacki, E.: The Essence and the Limits of Medical Knowledge (1899). In: Löwy, I. (ed.), pp. 50–57 (1991)

Chiffi, D., Pietarinen, A.V.: Fundamental uncertainty and values. Philosophia **45**(3), 1027–1037 (2017)

Federspil, G.: Logica clinica I principi del metodo in medicina. McGraw Hill, Milano (2004)

Federspil, G.: Spiegazione e causalità in medicina. Nuova Civiltà Delle Macchine **23**, 67–86 (2005)

Federspil, G.: Diagnosi. In: Pagnini, A. (ed.) Filosofia della medicina. Epistemologia, ontologia, etica, diritto, pp. 277–290. Carocci, Roma (2010)

Festa, R.: Principio di evidenza totale, decisioni cliniche ed Evidence Based Medicine. In: Federspil, G., Giaretta, P. (eds.) Forme della razionalià medica, pp. 47–82. Rubbettino, Soveria Mannelli (2004)

Hájek, A.: Probability, logic, and probability logic. In: Goble, L. (ed.) The Blackwell Companion to Logic, pp. 362–384. Blackwell, Oxford (2001)

Johansson, I., Lynøe, N.: Medicine & Philosophy. A Twenty-First Century Introduction. Ontos Verlag, Frankfurt (2008)

Jonsen, A., Toulmin, S.: The abuse of casuistry. A history of moral reasoning. Berkeley, CA: University of California Press Journals (1988).

Lagiou, P., Adami, H., Trichopoulos, D.: Causality in Cancer Epidemiology. Eur. J. Epidemiol. **20**(7), 565–574 (2005)

Löwy, I. (ed.): The Polish School of Philosophy of Medicine. From Tytus Chalubinski (1820–1889) to Ludwik Fleck (1896–1961). Kluwer Academic Publisher, Dordrecht (1991)

MeSH (Medical Subject Headings): Laryngeal Edema (2018) [The National Library of Medicine], retrieved from https://www.ncbi.nlm.nih.gov/mesh/68007819. Accessed 21.07.2020

Murri, A.: Quattro lezioni e una perizia. Il problema del metodo in medicina e biologia. Zanichelli, Bologna (1972)

Murri, A.: (2004). Dizionario di metodologia clinica. In: Baldini, M, Malavasi, A. (eds.) A. Delfino Editore, Roma (2004)

Reichenbach, H.: The Direction of Time. University of California Press, Berkeley and Los Angeles (1956)

Russo, F., Williamson, J.: Interpreting causality in the health sciences. Int. Stud. Philos. Sci. **21**(2), 157–170 (2007)

Salmon, W.C.: Probabilistic causality. Pac. Philos. Q. **61**(1–2), 50–74 (1980)

Scandellari, C., Federspil, G.: Metodologia medica. Edizioni L. Pozzi, Roma (1985)

Scandellari, C.: La metodologia in medicina. In: Pagnini, A. (ed.) Filosofia della medicina. Epistemologia, ontologia, etica, diritto, pp. 221–254. Carocci, Roma (2010)

Scriven, M.: Explanation and prediction in evolutionary theory. Science **130**, 477–482 (1959)

Slottje P., Sluijs J.P., van der Knol A.B.: Expert elicitation: methodological suggestions for its use in environmental health impact assessment. RIVM letter report 630004001/2008 (2008)

Suppes, P.: A Probabilistic Theory of Causality. North-Holland Publishing Company, Amsterdam (1970)

Uffink, J.: The principle of the common cause faces the Bernstein Paradox. Philos. Sci. **66**, S512–S525 (1999)

Weinstock, C.B., Goodenough, J.B., Klein, A.Z.: Measuring assurance case confidence using Baconian probabilities. In: 2013 1st international workshop on assurance cases for software-intensive systems (ASSURE), pp. 7–11. IEEE (2013)

Zanotti, R., Chiffi, D.: Diagnostic frameworks and nursing diagnoses: a normative stance. Nurs. Philos. **16**(1), 64–73 (2015)

Chapter 4
Clinical Hypotheses in Diagnostic and Prognostic Reasoning

4.1 Introduction

Hypotheses production is a central issue in clinical reasoning, both for diagnostic and prognostic judgments. In contrast to the strong scholarly interest in diagnosis, not much attention has been devoted so far to the notion of prognosis in the literature on the foundations of clinical reasoning.[1] Likely, the main reasons for this lie in the difficulty in applying taxonomical and formal models of prognosis to clinical activities, and in finding genuinely helpful prognostic guidelines to suit all the cases that clinicians encounter in their daily practice. Prognostication seems to be particularly sensitive to a physician's clinical expertise and expert opinion.[2] Expert clinicians are much more skilful in diagnostics than in forecasting (and communicating) their patients' future state of health (Christakis et al. 2000). Moreover, optimistic bias and anchoring are usually recognizable in clinicians' predictions.[3] Establishing a prognosis demands strong critical and logical reasoning skills in order to make sense of the complex methods needed to prognosticate soundly. This happens because the process of reaching a prognosis makes sense when it refers to a particular patient more than when it relies on mere population-based notions regarding the natural history

---

[1] A notable exception concerns the publications promoted by the PROGnosis RESearch Strategy (PROGRESS) Partnership on topics such as fundamental prognosis, prognostic factors, prognostic models and stratified medicine research https://progress-partnership.org/. The first of these publications provides an overview of the benefits of research on prognosis (Hemingway et al. 2013), like the fact that prognostic research may contribute to the generalizability of the results of clinical trials for specific populations.

[2] For an analytic discussion of the crucial role of expert opinions for clinical knowledge, see Tonelli (1999).

[3] Optimistic bias is seen, for instance, in the prognostication of terminally-ill patients (Christakis et al. 2000).

© The Editor(s) (if applicable) and The Author(s), under exclusive license
to Springer Nature Switzerland AG 2021
D. Chiffi, *Clinical Reasoning: Knowledge, Uncertainty, and Values in Health Care*,
Studies in Applied Philosophy, Epistemology and Rational Ethics 58,
https://doi.org/10.1007/978-3-030-59094-9_4

of a disease. The idiographic feature of prognosis is possibly one of the reasons why medicine still cannot be conceived as a strictly scientific discipline, but rather retains some of the characteristics of an art.

Applying population-based medical knowledge to arrive at an understanding of a particular clinical case is not always a direct process, even in presence of taxonomical tools. The Polish philosopher of medicine Wladyslaw Bieganski explained the classical view of the translation of medical knowledge as follows: "for us the term 'applied scientific discipline' means a discipline which applies the results obtained in the theoretical sciences to certain practical goals. It might be argued that such an application should not be considered as a science and we should not speak of applied sciences, but of the application of theoretical science to practice" (Bieganski 1908, p. 116). This approach comes close to the classical biomedical model of knowledge translation, according to which codified clinical knowledge gained at population level can be applied to a specific clinical case once the concerned patient has been assigned to a reference class.[4] According to this view, there is no place for emergent features of knowledge in clinical practice. This is, in fact, the typical situation in which the diagnostic process takes place. Clinicians have to *select* an already known hypothesis capable of explaining their patient's signs and symptoms, enabling them to identify a disease or syndrome. Matters are much more complicated in prognostics because emergent features of clinical knowledge and new clinical possibilities may shape the relationship between the prognosis and the real course of a disease in a given patient. Such complexity holds true since clinical knowledge is not always fixed but may dynamically evolve thanks to, for instance, new technologies or innovations. Emergentist aspects of clinical knowledge may consequently crop up, and this possibility may add to the uncertainty of a prognosis.[5] Bieganski made clear that what we have called "the classical model of knowledge translation" does not hold for clinical practice because "practice has its specific problems distinct from those in which theoretical science is engaged. These problems may be solved on the basis of the data supplied by the theoretical sciences, but the search for the solution is the subject of a specific kind of scientific research." (Bieganski 1908, p. 116). Solving such problems in clinical practice also calls for a way of thinking that be able to accommodate the specificities and fallibility of empirical hypotheses used in practice. I hold that logic, also in its abductive forms, may help physicians ground their diagnostic and prognostic reasoning with hypotheses, thereby enhancing their patients' health conditions.

I will defend the view that creative abduction, albeit being rarely involved in the diagnostic process (even if still possible[6]), is instead commonly used in the

---

[4]The identification of the reference class in a probabilistic explanation has been extensively analysed; see Hempel (1958) and Salmon (1970).

[5]On the distinction between the "cascade model" (that, in the clinical setting, can be seen as coinciding with the "classical biomedical model") and the "emergentist model" of knowledge translation, see Carrier (2010). For an analysis of the implications of the classical biomedical model, see Kirkengen et al. (2015).

[6]For instance, this is the case for the diagnosis of "Patient 1" of Covid19 in Italy. In this regard, see Chap. 1 and the Appendix of this book.

prognostic one. This is due to the fact that diagnosis is subject to the risk of error, meaning that the probability of taking a wrong decision is *computable* and *known*; whereas the prognostic judgment is often associated to *fundamental uncertainty*, i.e. the impossibility to compute probability when making a decision because some scenarios are, for instance, not predictable.

4.2 From Diagnosis to Prognosis

In this section I will explore some epistemological features related to the fallibilist dimension of hypotheses used in diagnosis and the nature of the uncertainty associated with them.

Before any therapy can be administered (which is the ultimate goal of clinical intervention), a patient's pathological condition has to be diagnosed. The diagnostic process comes across numerous issues, since in clinical practice it is very unusual to encounter a pathognomonic sign, i.e. specific, incontrovertible evidence of the presence of a particular disease. And diagnoses are rarely certain because they are a key element of clinical knowledge, whose empirical nature makes it inherently liable to various types of error (Hempel 1965). In the case of diagnostic tests, the inherent inductive risk is associated with the tests' false-positive and false-negative rates: neither types of error can be removed completely, so a diagnosis may be perfectly rational, but still wrong. Such important feature of diagnostics is sometimes overlooked in clinical practice. The risk of error is associated to a *known* probability regarding an uncertain situation. At least in line of principle, it is possible to compute the probability of making a wrong diagnosis given the available evidence, which represents a seminal feature of diagnostic reasoning.

In addition to its risk of error, a diagnosis has to be seen as having a temporal dimension (Chiffi and Zanotti 2015). As Miettinen and Flegel put it, "illness at any given diagnosis along its course has not only its basic nature and current particulars as well as its future course; it also has its past (its history of pathologic development)" (Miettinen and Flegel 2003, p. 334). Although many different types of clinical diagnosis can be established,[7] diagnoses—as we have seen—can be classified in two broad categories: *nosographic* and *pathophysiological* (Federspil 2004). The former aim to assign a patient's pathological condition to a specific category with a nosographic taxonomy. In point of fact, recognizing the causes, explanations and mechanisms behind the individual's pathological state is not tantamount to formulating a nosographic diagnosis.[8] Pathophysiological diagnoses, instead, focus specifically on the past to shed light on how a patient's disease developed, and thus explain his or her pathological condition. Hence, an essential characteristic setting apart pathophysiological diagnoses is the requirement of explanations.

---

[7]On the logical reconstruction of some key features of diagnoses, see Chiffi and Zanotti (2015).

[8]Of course, the selection of the categories within a taxonomy may or may not be guided by causes or explanations.

Explanations, in fact, are needed when we do not have thorough knowledge of a phenomenon. And to make every explanation valid, each one must be empirically confirmable by means of logical or probabilistic laws. Before formulating an explanation, it is important to clarify the meaning of the terms involved, replacing any vague term (*explicandum*) with a more precise one (the *explicatum*)—a method called "explication". According to Carnap (1950), in a good explication the *explicatum* must: (a) be similar to the *explicandum*; (b) be clearly defined, formalized and inserted in the context of a scientific theory; (c) be a fruitful concept, i.e. it may follow from nomological statements (in the case of empirical theories) or logical theorems (in the case of logical concepts); and (d) be simple. Given that any pathophysiological diagnosis requires explanations, and any explanation can be grounded on the explication of the terms involved, it follows that a pathophysiological diagnosis may be refined by an explication. In other words, before attempting any semeiotic interpretation of a patient's medical history, signs and symptoms, laboratory data, and so forth, clinicians should try to adopt a rigorous scientific terminology (and methodology) in order to arrive at a synthesis of the patient's set of signs and symptoms (or '*syndromic complex*'[9] in the language of special pathology). At this point, clinical hypotheses that might explain some of a patient's pathological features are conceived or selected, examined and compared, and interpreted for diagnostic purposes. All these steps, however, are not often possible in diagnostics, and clinicians have to develop some strategies in order to cope with this fact.

The procedure, called *differential diagnosis*, requires to take into consideration a precise, finite set of hypotheses and then rule some of them out. A differential diagnosis may be formulated to identify a particular hypothesis, even when there is no saying for sure that that hypothesis is right (for instance, it may not have been among the hypotheses originally considered). Alternatively, if evidence emerges to confirm one of the original hypotheses, then a differential diagnosis may establish the presence of one disease and rule out the possibility of others. A set of empirical data can logically confute not just a proposition expressing a single hypothesis, but a whole set of propositions. This phenomenon is known as *epistemological holism*; it holds that, when a false conclusion is reached in an argument, it is logically impossible to establish which of the premises of the argument is (or are) false (Duhem 1991). Intuitively, starting from the truth of the premises of a deductive argument and applying a sound rule of inference, we find that every inferable conclusion is 'atomistically' true. It is, in fact, well-known that deductive logic is truth-preserving. Conversely, given a false conclusion, the falsity applies holistically to the whole set of premises used in the argument. The premises used in clinical arguments are generally based on hypotheses as well as initial conditions, physiological laws, etc., so a falsity deriving from clinical data cannot but affect the whole set of premises, and not just a single one expressing a given hypothesis. This means that a hypothesis cannot be safely ruled out in a deductive framework when it is associated with other

---

[9] A syndromic complex is the association of patient's signs and symptoms with a cluster of diagnostic hypotheses (Federspil and Vettor 1999).

conditions, whereas adopting an inductive framework enables us to compute and assess the impact of different hypotheses on available data (Feinstein 1977).

Within the philosophy of science various scientific explanatory models that are relevant to the pathophysiological diagnostic process have been proposed. Some of the more common are:

1. the *nomological-deductive* model, in which a conclusion (the *explanandum*) can be derived deductively from the *explanans*, which consists of general laws and initial conditions. The logical constraints of this model are as follows: the *explanandum* must be a logical consequence of the *explanans*; the *explanans* must contain at least a general law and express empirical content. A further empirical constraint requires that the *explanans* consist of true statements.
2. the *statistical-inductive model*, in which the *explanans* consists of statistical laws and initial conditions, and the *explanandum* is derivable from the *explanans* with a given degree of probability.
3. *teleological* (or *functional*) *explanations*, which usually take the following form: the function A in a system S with an organization C is to enable S in an environment E to engage in a process P. Teleological explanations are often used in the biomedical sciences, and their structure is such that they explain phenomena by taking the specific goals of biological mechanisms into account.[10]

When there is an explanation for the phenomenon being investigated, a pathophysiological diagnosis may be established. In other words, no pathophysiological diagnosis can be formulated in the event of medically inexplicable symptoms. On the other hand, a nosographic diagnosis can, in principle, be formulated on the basis of unexplained symptoms, since they have a signalling value recognizable within a nosographic category. This is the case of, among others, many autoimmune diseases.

The information provided by a diagnosis enables the therapeutic options and various clinical issues to be analysed.[11] This is the point where a prognosis can be established, within a process that is highly sensitive to many individual factors associated with a given patient, and to some emergent features of knowledge in a particular clinical setting.[12] For that reason, prognostication is often associated to fundamental uncertainty, and not just to a risk of error in which the probability of a specific event may be known.

---

[10]Other explanatory models are available, e.g. statistical deductive models, mechanistic ones, etc. We do not discuss all the main features of such models here because we are only interested in their role in diagnostic and prognostic reasoning.

[11]On the notion of clinical possibility, see Chiffi and Zanotti (2016).

[12]It is worth noting that the 'anticipatory' dimension of medicine is increasingly based on genetic research, and is associated not only with epistemic, but also with ethical and cultural aspects.

4.3   Foundations of Prognostication

Prognostication is an action that has been somewhat left on the sidelines of current medical practice (Rich 2001). A prognosis is the end-result of a fundamental clinical assessment that focuses mainly on the future, which is why it is considered more difficult than establishing diagnoses or making treatment decisions (Christakis and Sachs 1996). Even when a diagnosis has been soundly formulated, the prognosis may be uncertain because our understanding of pathological conditions is always incomplete, and diseases may develop in unpredictable ways (Austoni and Federspil 1975). This means that prognostic judgment faces fundamental uncertainty (also known as 'Keynesian uncertainty') (Keynes 2008), since probability measures can hardly be assigned to specific future events that shape such type of judgment. In fact, relevant prognostic information may not be available when formulating a prognosis, decreasing, therefore, the potential to predict the patient's disease course. Despite this remarkable fact, prognostics is still based on the concept of risk, a notion that may be used in the context of *certainty of uncertainty*, but not in the context of *fundamental uncertainty*.

The aim of prognostics is traditionally to judge: (i) the duration of a future disease stage in a given patient (*prognosi quoad tempus*); (ii) the probability of a patient recovering from a disease (*prognosi quoad veletudinem*); or (iii) the chances of a patient's survival (*prognosi quoad vitam*) (Rizzi 1993). All these types of prognosis are made with a margin of uncertainty, being a prognosis usually formulated as the *probability* of an outcome and/or of a patient's health taking a certain course (in terms of a particular disease) within a specified time interval (Djulbegovic et al. 2011; Miettinen 2011). Yet, this classical view on prognostication makes substantial use of the notions of probability and risk, despite the fact this may be unsuitable when dealing with fundamental uncertainty. Moreover, also the latter type of uncertainty has some cognitive and emotional factors associated with patient's expectations. Patients may, for instance, experience fear of knowing their future.[13]

From the patients' point of view, having to ignore or cope with severe and fundamental uncertainty about their future health is psychologically harmful (Smith et al.

---

[13]When a prognosis is very poor, physicians may prefer not to inform their patients. Physicians tend to consider such a prognosis as a self-fulfilling prophecy, because it is usually believed to occur in association with clinical treatments or placebo (or nocebo) effects (Christakis 1999; Rich 2002). A self-fulfilling prophecy is a prediction which induces a person believing in it to behave in such a way that makes it ultimately come true. In the case of prognostics, the core idea is that being informed of a poor prognosis can have a negative effect on a patient's future health. The impression that this might play a part in the relations between physician and patient is questionable in such a multi-agent context as the clinical one, however. Seen from Lewis's perspective (Lewis 1975), in a multi-agent context, self-fulfilling beliefs require higher-order beliefs to justify them, combined with higher beliefs (or ideally common knowledge) shared by different epistemic agents. Such conditions are typically violated in the sphere of prognostics because of the asymmetry of information between physician and patient (Chiffi and Zanotti 2017). Prognostic beliefs can therefore hardly be considered as self-fulfilling, since they occur in a multi-agent context, where there may not exist converging higher beliefs for the patient and the physician. This being the case, physicians' concerns about communicating a prognosis to patients often seem to be unwarranted.

2013). Patients' hopes and expectations are based on higher-order beliefs concerning the prognostic information they receive from their doctors. To give an example, the famous biologist Stephen J. Gould survived 20 years after being told that the median survival rate for patients with an abdominal mesothelioma like his was eight months. His case suggests how population-based statistics cannot predict what will happen in a specific case, a fact that should always be borne in mind when giving patients prognostic information (Gould 2002).

If, however, doctors were to come up with a wrong prognosis, they may negatively affect not only their patient's health, but, also their own professional credibility. From this point we can see why prognostic accuracy can be so frustrating, especially since predicting a patient's future health conditions is by no means easy.

Not all facets of prognostics are sensitive to doctors' and patients' beliefs. A prognosis is also influenced by *prognostic markers* (which are unmodifiable and uninfluenced by the course of the disease) and *prognostic factors* (which are modifiable and dependent on how the disease develops). Prognostic markers and factors include: (i) the stage and severity of a pathological condition associated with a disease; (ii) an individual's resistance to disease[14]; (iii) a patient's gender and age; (iv) a patient's preferences on treatments, living environment, behaviour, and so forth (Wiesemann 1998; Del Mar et al. 2008). Elucidating the relationships between general and specific cases can be quite complicated, especially from a prognostic standpoint. There is no standardized or mechanistic way to correlate a new patient to the results obtained from samples of other patients with the same disease (Hilden and Habbema 1987; Thorne and Sawatzky 2014). Moreover, given the fundamental uncertainty of prognostication, the set of prognostic factors may be incomplete or loosely clinically significant.

Like diagnoses, prognoses include a temporal factor as they are likely to change over time. They can be classified within two main categories: *nosographic* and *pathophysiological* (Federspil 2004). A *nosographic prognosis* is based on a nosographic diagnosis and aims to predict when patients will reach a certain future stage of their disease. This prediction is based on statistical probabilities elicited from population-based data. On the other hand, a *pathophysiological prognosis* is based on a pathophysiological diagnosis, meaning that the prediction of a future stage of disease in a given patient is in this case grounded on knowledge of the explanation for his or her disease. Intuitively, if the initial condition occurs before a clinical judgment is established, then we have an explanation; if not, we have a prediction (as in the case of prognosis). Given the level of uncertainty inherent to medical knowledge, prognostic explanations do not usually involve universal laws, another reason why the concept of prognosis is not deterministic (Sadegh-Zadeh 2012).

Especially in the case of pathophysiological prognoses, knowing the probability of a disease stage occurring at population level may often be held as scarcely relevant to a specific patient, since patient-related factors can profoundly affect prognostication.

---

[14]Individual variability, in terms of patients' different predisposition to health and disease, was the focus of the research program at the Padua School of Constitutional Medicine organized at the beginning of the twentieth century by Achille De Giovanni. See De Giovanni (1909).

But another source of uncertainty is also present in clinical practice: not all aspects of a given explanation are always reported in detail. Some pathophysiological laws may not be explicitly stated, for instance, leading to partial explanations that are usually termed "incomplete" or "elliptic". A full explanation may instead be provided in a rational reconstruction once all the constituent parts of the explanation have been produced (Hempel 1962). When doctors only count with very patchy explanations and limited information, their prognostic judgment can be suspended waiting for further signs to emerge in the natural history of the disease. It is occasionally possible to infer a simple prognosis from the identification of a patient's signs and symptoms alone. The level of uncertainty of any prognosis—partly due to the inherent difficulty of foreseeing the course a disease in a particular patient—makes it reasonable to assume that some hypotheses (formulated in the light of a diagnosis) may not make sense of what is happening to a patient's health, and may thus need to be reconsidered. In this case, new hypotheses (not taken into account during the initial diagnostic workup) may be formulated, leading to an adjustment of the original diagnosis.

Finally, a prognosis is shaped by the therapeutic options available for a given condition. Physicians predict the future course of a disease based on the alleged efficacy of the treatment chosen for a given patient. After reviewing all the subsequent stages of the patient's clinical management, doctors should ideally arrive at a final retrospective assessment (*epicrisis*) of all possible diagnostic, prognostic or treatment errors.

4.4   Abduction in Diagnostic and Prognostic Reasoning

Abductive reasoning has been recognized as an essential tool in the clinical setting. According to Upshur, "inferences in clinical medicine made on the basis of statistical models and clinical encounters are characteristically abductive. They should be regarded as tentative statements that the inference holds, is provisionally the case, or pragmatically justifies action" (Upshur 1997, p. 204). Both the justification and the growth of our medical knowledge can be analysed using the concept of abduction, which may very well serve the purpose of grounding our clinical reasoning. The most common type of inference is abductive inference, having the best applicability (in contrast to the deductive and inductive types) in diagnostics since judgements can be made based on the available information, even if incomplete. It is usually assumed that abductive inference is, in a narrow sense, the only ampliative form of reasoning.

The following justifications are usually acknowledged by parties making abductive inferences. It is generally assumed that: (i) an unexpected and interesting observation stems from the premises of an abductive inference; and (ii) there is an increase in the initial plausibility of the hypothesis expressed in the conclusion of the abductive inference. In deductive logic, from the (certainty of the) truth of a premise we can infer the (certainty of the) truth of the conclusion. In abductive inferences, on the other hand, conclusions (expressing hypotheses) can only be plausible.

The use of abductive inference has been recognized in medicine. An example of abductive inference in medicine is outlined below, drawn from the study by Auguste Loubatières on the mechanism associated with hypoglycemic sulfonamides:

1. In patients suffering from typhoid and treated with 2254RP the administration of this drug causes hypoglycemia.
2. If the drug stimulates the endocrine pancreas to produce insulin, then the onset of hypoglycemia is a matter of course.
3. There is reason to suspect that the hypothesis that the drug stimulates the endocrine pancreas to produce insulin is true (Federspil 2004).

More specifically, hypothetical reasoning in the form of abduction finds many applications in medicine and nursing within diagnostic, prognostic and therapeutic settings (Bissessur et al. 2009). Decision making is an important part of the diagnostic process, specifically when it comes to choosing the most adequate hypotheses to identify a patient's disease (from among a finite number of known hypotheses consistent with pathological knowledge), and to prescribing the most appropriate treatment in light of the prediction of the future course of the patient's condition. According to the philosopher Charles Sanders Peirce, abduction differs from either induction or deduction, and can be formulated as follows:

The surprising fact, C, is observed.

But if A were true, C would be a matter of course.

Hence, there is reason to suspect that A is true. (Peirce 1931, CP 5.189)[15]

The above cited abductive arguments are among the most famous from Peirce's writings, although more analytic ones can be found. Abduction cannot be applied to classical deduction, which is a logical system where truth is transmitted with certainty from the premises to the conclusion. Peirce saw abduction as a logical procedure that holds also in what we now call the 'context of discovery', that is, in the genesis of a scientific theory. Moreover, logical reasoning is nowadays also part

---

[15]On Peirce and the notion of abduction, see Paavola (2005) and Pietarinen and Bellucci (2014). As masterfully acknowledged by Woods (2013), Peirce's "important ideas" on abduction are the following: (P0) Abduction is triggered by surprise. (P1) Abduction is a form of guessing. Since we are rather remarkably good at guessing, it can only be supposed that we are likewise rather good at abducing. (P2) A successful abduction provides no grounds for believing the abduced proposition to be true. (P3) Rather than believing them, the proper thing to do with abduced hypotheses is to send them off to experimental trial (CP 5.599, 6.469–6.473, 7.202–219). (P4) The connection between the truth of the abduced hypothesis and the observed fact is subjunctive (CP 5.189). (P5) The inference that the abduction licenses is not to the proposition H, but rather that H's truth is something that might plausibly be conjectured (CP 5.189). (P6) The "hence" of the Peircean conclusion is ventured defeasibly (CP 5.189). See Peirce (1931). Peirce's seminal intuitions are the guiding ideas of the Gabbay-Woods (GW) schema of abduction (Gabbay and Woods 2006). A pragmatic interpretation and a semi-formalization of this schema have been provided in Chiffi and Pietarinen (2020a, b). The GW schema was introduced as a refinement of the AKM model of abduction. In the acronym AKM, A refers to Aliseda (1998, 2005), K to Kowalski (1979), Kuipers (1999), and Kakas et al. (1992), M to Magnani (2009) and Meheus et al. (2002). In Magnani (2009) it is also presented his eco-cognitive model of abduction. For an analysis of Magnani's views on abduction, see Park (2017).

of the 'context of justification' of a theory. Unfortunately, after Peirce, abduction in the context of justification (AJ) has often been portrayed as a possible form of 'inference to the best explanation of a theory', i.e. an inference that is justified by the hypothesis judged most adequate to explain a given phenomenon. Still, abduction and inference to the best explanation should not be confused, since there is no guarantee that an abducted hypothesis is the best explanation. AJ plays an essential role in the medical diagnostic process, viz. when a selection is made from among a finite set of hypotheses that are justified by pathological and scientific knowledge[16] (Barosi et al. 1983). Abduction in the context of discovery (AD), on the other side, is also acknowledged as a sort of heuristic principle which orientates the adoption of some 'hypothesis-candidate', namely, statements that are not positively confirmed by the evidence but whose negation is unjustified (not proved). Doctors have to select a working hypothesis from among a given finite set of possible hypotheses codified by clinical knowledge in order to make sense of a patient's anamnestic cues. AD is more often employed by nurses, however, because a nursing diagnosis has a less codified epistemological dimension and is more likely to be associated with conditions for which 'there is no previously established principle or cause that explains the observed surprising phenomenon' (Stanley and Campos 2013). Nursing diagnosis aims to find new hypothesis-candidates in order to orientate the provision of services and patient care.

According to Frankfurt (1958) an explanatory hypothesis A always has to be acknowledged before the conclusion of the abductive argument, implying that abduction cannot be very creative. He in fact made the point in contrast to Peirce that, more than creating new hypotheses, abduction rather works as a filter in the adoption of good hypothesis-candidates for testing. However, hypothesis A in the major premise and conclusion of the abductive schema have different modes, since A in the premise is the antecedent of the subjunctive conditional, while in the conclusion is put as an invitation to investigate further A (a "co-hortative" mood) (Anderson 1986; Ma and Pietarinen 2018). The conclusion is "a good working hypothesis to go ahead with, at least as a basis for conducting tests or, if tests are not necessary, as a basis for provisional action or inaction" (Walton 2004, p. 144). The major role of abduction is thus to help us select hypotheses in the context of justification, and to select hypothesis-candidates in the context of the discovery[17] (Douven 2011).

If we reframe Peirce's general structure of abductive inference according to a classical deductive logic, then we stumble upon the fallacy of affirming the consequence, while struggling to reformulate the above argument properly in an inductive

---

[16]Since testing hypotheses is time, energy and money consuming, Peirce proposed a methodology called "economy of research" in order to evaluate different research proposal based on their costs and potential benefits. See Chiffi et al. (2020).

[17]In nursing, abduction should serve in this function of selecting hypothesis-candidates with a view to improving health care paths. In fact, there is no precise and codified scientific framework for nursing knowledge, contrary to what happens in medical diagnostics, which is based on the methods and results of many different sciences. Some possible limitations of abductive reasoning applied to nursing, like those presented in Råholm (2010) for instance, are investigated by Lipscomb (2012).

framework.[18] The fact C is observed and is surprising in the light of an accepted set of explicative hypotheses concerning C; a set which we can call Hs. A new candidate of explanatory hypothesis A would elucidate the onset of C better than would be the case if the initial set of hypotheses were left unchanged. It thus follows that hypothesis A is strengthened. Of course, this is not a conclusive argument, but merely a plausible one. It is worth noting that A is not contained in the set Hs, meaning that: (i) A had not been conceived previously, i.e. no explicative function for phenomena like C was attributed to A, and A was now merely being *selected* from among other hypotheses to make sense of C; or (ii) A was *created* because of the difficulty of explaining C by means of Hs. In both cases, there may be reason to suspect that A is true. The status of selected or created (clinical) hypothesis in abduction is critically investigated in Thagard (1992, 2006), Magnani (1997, 2001, 2009), Ramoni et al. (1992).[19] The distinction between creative and selective abduction was firstly described in Magnani (2001).

In the clinical activity of diagnostics, hypotheses are merely selected from an existing set of possible options. Clinicians have to identify and isolate a hypothesis for testing (possibly by means of abductive inferences) in order to arrive at a diagnosis for a given patient. Strictly speaking, it is very unlikely that a *creation* of objective clinical knowledge occurs in the diagnostic process (Murri 1972). This does not mean that diagnostic hypotheses associated with specific signs and symptoms remain fixed: they may evolve in the light of therapeutic and prognostic considerations, though they ideally remain finite and may be encoded again in a new diagnostic framework.

Stanley and Campos take a different stance on the creative/selective nature of hypotheses in diagnostic reasoning (Stanley and Campos 2013, 2016), arguing for a balance between the generation and the selection of hypotheses in medical diagnostics. Criticism to their view may stem from the interpretation given to the nature of the accepted set of explicative hypotheses (Hs). On the one hand, if Hs is relativized to the set of hypotheses that the physician associates with C, then we might say that hypotheses could be created in the abductive process grounded on diagnostic reasoning. However, a physician may also be unaware of a relevant explicative hypothesis for C, in which case there can be no creation of hypotheses, but only the physician's lack of knowledge. When the set of Hs is interpreted objectively, a "creative" production of hypotheses in clinical diagnostics is unlikely (in a narrow sense) because it seldom happens to assess and recognize a pathological condition that has not been already somewhat described or codified. Instead, it is possible to assume that "when facing atypical or complex cases, physicians may have to combine their knowledge of possible diseases in novel ways to explain the condition of that specific patient" (Stanley and Campos 2016). It follows that knowledge about known diseases can be merged and codified in order to develop new diagnostic patterns for more complex situations.

---

[18]For a critical analysis of the forms of induction, deduction and abduction in clinical reasoning, see Festa et al. (2009).

[19]For an interesting historical application of abduction to Akkadian medical diagnosis, see Barés Gómez (2018).

That no new hypotheses are usually created by the diagnostic judgment process suggests it is not common to create objective medical knowledge in an ordinary case of clinical reasoning. This view may be particularly challenged, instead, if one focuses on the role of hypotheses in prognostic judgments. It is plausible to assume that creative forms of abduction cannot be readily dismissed when formulating a prognosis because the initial set of hypotheses to consider cannot be easily restricted. There are numerous hypothetical factors (of an environmental, genetic or behavioural nature) capable of shaping the prognostic judgment and contributing to its fundamental uncertainty.[20] In formulating a prognosis, the most difficult task is to make sense of the extreme uncertainty regarding the individual disease pathway. Such uncertainty may push the physician to generate new explicative hypotheses or little explored scenarios.

On the other hand, the conceivability of a prognostic hypothesis is usually improved by clinical expertise, in particular when a prognosis is intended to be grounded on specific pathophysiological explanations. Hence, clinicians encounter emerging aspects of clinical knowledge and new hypotheses. In this light, medicine is not merely an applied science like "applied mathematics" because abstract and general knowledge cannot be applied directly to a particular clinical context. It is during the prognostication process that a synthesis can be achieved from the interplay between encoded knowledge and the hypotheses emerging from a given clinical context.[21] Emergent hypotheses with a potential explicative power regarding a pathological condition in a patient may prompt a review of the main steps involved in a clinical judgment. It is on the prognostic level, moreover, that a patient's decisions and values may influence the physician's clinical reasoning. The generation of new prognostic hypotheses is often a good strategy for dealing with the uncertainty of the future course of the disease. It is therefore important to investigate the nature of diagnostic and prognostic hypotheses based on their different role in abductive inferences.

4.5   Conclusions

Patients are usually extremely keen to receiving accurate prognostic information. Predictions of their future health conditions may prompt or enable patients to make significant decisions concerning their lives. For all its importance, the notion of prognosis has yet to receive an adequate degree of philosophical and foundational attention, which may be due to the difficulties inherent in accurate prognostics. In the

---

[20] As stated before, prognostic hypotheses regard future health conditions. Hypotheses on infinite or unsurveyable domains, as the one given by future times, express sentences not in principle decidable (Dummett 1976). In virtues of this, prognostic hypotheses are extremely difficult to be tested and codified. On the contrary, since diagnostic hypotheses involve a present health condition, they might be decidable, at least in line of principle.

[21] Of course, also non-epistemic aspects of clinical reasoning such as ethical and social values play a non-secondary role in shaping the clinical context (Risjord 2011).

light of these considerations, a considerable body of critical thinking on the topic of prognostication was discussed, pointing out the distinction between nosographic and pathophysiological types of diagnosis and prognosis, whilst stressing the importance of the explication and explanation processes. I have pointed out and discussed the fact that pathophysiological diagnoses and prognoses require suitable explanatory models. The chapter also covered the *certainty of uncertainty* related to the (probabilistic) risk of error for diagnostic reasoning as well as the fundamental uncertainty associated to prognostication. Then, I have distinguished between different forms of hypothetical reasoning for the purpose of diagnostic and prognostic judgments. Hypotheses in the diagnostic framework are usually selected from among an existing set of initial hypotheses; and, in general, no new hypotheses are created. On the other hand, I have argued that reasoning with hypotheses in prognostics may also be a creative process, since new prognostic strategies may be created in order to deal with the fundamental uncertainty of prognostic judgment. Classical prognostic reasoning based on probabilistic risk analysis may indeed face significant limitations in its application, since it is based on the notion of risk instead of fundamental uncertainty. In prognostics, fundamental uncertainty may in fact be methodologically challenging when in presence of nosographic prognosis, since even the nature of a pathophysiological mechanism associated to the onset of a disease may be unknown.

I explored how abductive inferences may contribute to developing a new approach towards the fundamental uncertainty often involved in prognostication. Moreover, emergent and individualized clinical features (based on patients' attitudes and values) can substantially affect their prognosis, which explains why prognostication always focuses on individual patients (and also why the notion of the natural history of a disease is overall weak). Subsequently, I have clarified the distinction between the selective and creative dimensions of clinical hypotheses used in diagnostics and prognostics with different forms of abduction.

My analysis underscores the limitations of the classical biomedical model of knowledge transfer according to which population-based knowledge can be applied directly to a single patient. It supports some aspects of the emergentist model of knowledge translation (Carrier 2010) in medicine (that I will discuss in some of the subsequent chapters), whereby epistemic novelties may emerge for the hypothetical reasoning not by virtue of the diagnostic judgment, but because of the prognostic judgment on a patient's future health conditions. Indeed, abduction can significantly contribute to clinical reasoning in the uncertainty of judging both present and future of ongoing diseases.

References

Aliseda, A.: Seeking Explanations: Abduction in Logic Philosophy of Science and Artificial Intelligence. Stanford University Press, Stanford (1998)

Aliseda, A.: The logic of abduction in the light of Peirce's pragmatism. Semiotica **153**(1/4), 363–374 (2005)

Anderson, D.R.: The evolution of Peirce's concept of abduction. Trans. Charles S. Peirce Soc. **22**(2), 145–164 (1986)

Austoni, M., Federspil, G.: Principi di metodologia clinica. Cedam, Padova (1975)

Barés Gómez, C.: Abduction in Akkadian medical diagnosis. J. Appl. Logics IfCoLog J. Logics Appl. **5**(8), 1697–1722 (2018)

Barosi, G., Magnani, L., Stefanelli, M.: Medical diagnostic reasoning: epistemological modeling as a strategy for design of computer-based consultation programs. Theoret. Med. **14**, 43–65 (1983)

Bieganski, W.: The logic of medicine or the critique of medical knowledge. In: Löwy, I. (ed.) The Polish School of Philosophy of Medicine. From Tytus Chalubinski (1820–1889) to Ludwik Fleck (1896–1961), pp. 112–120. Kluwer, Dordrecht (1990, original text 1908)

Bissessur, S.W., Geijteman, E.C.T., Al-Dulaimy, M., Teunissen, P.W., Richir, M.C., Arnold, A.E.R., de Vries, T.P.G.M.: Therapeutic reasoning: from hiatus to hypothetical model. J. Eval. Clin. Pract. **15**, 985–989 (2009)

Carnap, R.: Logical Foundations of Probability. University of Chicago Press, Chicago (1950)

Carrier, M.: Theories for use: on the bearing of basic science on practical problems. In: Suárez, M., Dorato, M., Rédei, M. (eds.) EPSA. Epistemology and Methodology of Science. Launch of the European Philosophy of Science Association, pp. 23–33. Springer, Dordrecht (2010)

Chiffi, D., Pietarinen, A.V.: Abduction within a pragmatic framework. Synthese **197**(6), 2507–2523 (2020a)

Chiffi, D., Pietarinen, A.-V.: The extended Gabbay-Woods schema and scientific practices. In: Gabbay, D., Magnani, L., Park, W., Pietarinen, A.-V. (eds.) Natural Arguments. A Tribute to John Woods. College Publications, London (2020b)

Chiffi, D., Zanotti, R.: Medical and nursing diagnoses: a critical comparison. J. Eval. Clin. Pract. **21**(1), 1–6 (2015)

Chiffi, D., Zanotti, R.: Perspectives on clinical possibility: elements of analysis. J. Eval. Clin. Pract. **22**(4), 509–514 (2016)

Chiffi, D., Zanotti, R.: Knowledge and belief in placebo effect. J. Med. Philos. **42**(1), 70–85 (2017)

Chiffi, D., Pietarinen, A.V., Proover, M.: Anticipation, abduction and the economy of research: the normative stance. Futures **115**, 102471 (2020)

Christakis, N.A.: Prognostication and bioethics. Daedalus **128**(4), 197–214 (1999)

Christakis, N.A., Sachs, G.A.: The role of prognosis in clinical decision-making. J. Gen. Intern. Med. **11**(7), 422–425 (1996)

Christakis, N.A., Smith, J.L., Parkes, C.M., Lamont, E.B.: Extent and determinants of error in doctors' prognoses in terminally ill patients: prospective cohort study. BMJ **320**(7233), 469–473 (2000)

De Giovanni, A.: The Morphology of the Human Body. Rebman Limited, London (1909)

Del Mar, C., Doust, J., Glasziou, P.P.: Clinical Thinking: Evidence, Communication and Decision Making. Wiley, Malden, Massachusetts (2008)

Djulbegovic, B., Hozo, I., Greenland, S.: Uncertainty in clinical medicine. In: Gifford, F. (ed.) Philosophy of Medicine. Handbook of the Philosophy of Science, vol. 16, pp. 299–356. Elsevier, Amsterdam (2011)

Douven, I.: Abduction. In: Stanford Encyclopedia of Philosophy. Available at: https://plato.stanford.edu/entries/abduction/index.html (2011). Accessed 20 July 2020

Duhem, P.: The Aim and Structure of Physical Theory. Princeton University Press, Princeton (1991)

Dummett, M.: What is a theory of meaning? (II). In: Evans, G., McDowell, J. (eds) Truth and Meaning: Essays in Semantics, pp. 67–137. Clarendon Press, Oxford (1976)

Federspil, G.: Logica Clinica. McGraw-Hill, Milan (2004)

Federspil, G., Vettor, R.: Clinical and laboratory logic. Clin. Chim. Acta **280**(1), 25–34 (1999)

Feinstein, A.R.: Clinical Biostatistics. Mosby, St. Louis (1977)

Festa, R., Crupi, V., Giaretta, P.: Deduzione, induzione e abduzione nelle scienze mediche. Logic Philos. Sci. **7**(1), 41–68 (2009)

Frankfurt, H.: Peirce's notion of abduction. J. Philos. **55**, 593–596 (1958)

Gabbay, D.M., Woods, J.: Advice on abductive logic. Logic J. IGPL **14**(2), 189–219 (2006)

Gould, S.J.: The median isn't the message. In: CancerGuide: Statistics. https://cancerguide.org/med ian_not_msg.html (2002). Accessed 20 July 2020

Hemingway, H., Croft, P., Perel, P., Hayden, J.A., Abrams, K., Timmis, A., Schroter, S., Altman, D.G., Riley, R.D., PROGRESS Group: Prognosis research strategy (PROGRESS) 1: a framework for researching clinical outcomes. BMJ **346**, e5595 (2013)

Hempel, C.G.: The theoretician's dilemma. In: Feigl, H., Scriven, M., Maxwell, G. (eds.) Minnesota Studies in the Philosophy of Science, vol. II, pp. 37–98. University of Minnesota Press, Minneapolis (1958)

Hempel, C.G.: Explanation in science and history. In: Colodny, R.C. (ed.) Frontiers of Science and Philosophy, pp. 9–19. The University of Pittsburgh Press, Pittsburgh (1962)

Hempel, C.G.: Science and human values. In: Aspects of Scientific Explanation and Other Essays in the Philosophy of Science, pp. 81–96. The Free Press, New York (1965)

Hilden, J., Habbema, J.D.F.: Prognosis in medicine: an analysis of its meaning and roles. Theoret. Med. **8**(3), 349–365 (1987)

Kakas, A., Kowalski, R.A., Toni, F.: Abductive logic programming. J. Log. Comput. **2**(6), 719–770 (1992)

Keynes, J.M.: The General Theory of Employment, Interest, and Money. Atlantic Publishers, New Delhi (2008, originally published in 1936)

Kirkengen, A.L., Ekeland, T.J., Getz, L., Hetlevik, I., Schei, E., Ulvestad, E., Vetlesen, A.J.: Medicine's perception of reality—a split picture: critical reflections on apparent anomalies within the biomedical theory of science. J. Eval. Clin. Pract. **22**(4), 496–501 (2015)

Kowalski, R.A.: Logic for Problem Solving. Elsevier, New York (1979)

Kuipers, T.A.F.: Abduction aiming at empirical progress of even truth approximation leading to a challenge for computational modelling. Found. Sci. **4**(3), 307–323 (1999)

Lewis, D.: Language and languages. In: Gunderson, K. (ed.) Minnesota Studies in the Philosophy of Science, vol. VII, pp. 3–35. University of Minnesota Press, Minneapolis (1975)

Lipscomb, M.: Abductive reasoning and qualitative research. Nurs. Philos. **13**(4), 244–256 (2012)

Ma, M., Pietarinen, A.V.: Let us investigate! Dynamic conjecture-making as the formal logic of abduction. J. Philos. Logic **47**(6), 913–945 (2018)

Magnani, L.: Basic science reasoning and clinical reasoning intertwined: epistemological analysis and consequences for medical education. Adv. Health Sci. Educ. **2**(2), 115–130 (1997)

Magnani, L.: Abduction, Reason and Science. Springer, Dordrecht (2001)

Magnani, L.: Abductive Cognition. The Epistemological and Eco-Cognitive Dimensions of Hypothetical Reasoning. Springer, Berlin-Heidelberg (2009)

Meheus, J., Verhoeven, L., Van Dyck, M., Provijn, D.: Ampliative adaptive logics and the foundation of logic-based approaches to abduction. In: Magnani, L., Nersessian, N.J., Pizzi, C. (eds.) Logical and Computational Aspects of Model-Based Reasoning, pp. 39–71. Kluwer Academic Publishers, Dordrecht (2002)

Miettinen, O.S.: Epidemiological Research: Terms and Concepts. Springer, Dordrecht (2011)

Miettinen, O.S., Flegel, K.M.: Elementary concepts of medicine: VIII. Knowing about a client's health: gnosis. J. Eval. Clin. Pract. **9**(3), 333–335 (2003)

Murri, A.: Quattro lezioni e una perizia. Il problema del metodo in medicina e biologia. Zanichelli, Bologna (1972)

Paavola, S.: Peircean abduction: instinct or inference? Semiotica **153**(1/4), 131–154 (2005)

Park, W.: Abduction in Context: The Conjectural Dynamics of Scientific Reasoning. Springer, Dordrecht (2017)

Peirce, C.S.: Collected Papers, vol. V. Harvard University Press, Cambridge, MA (1931). Cited as CP followed by volume and paragraph number

Pietarinen, A.V., Bellucci, F.: New light on Peirce's conceptions of retroduction, deduction, and scientific reasoning. Int. Stud. Philos. Sci. **28**(4), 353–373 (2014)

Råholm, M.B.: Abductive reasoning and the formation of scientific knowledge within nursing research. Nurs. Philos. **11**(4), 260–270 (2010)

Ramoni, M., Stefanelli, M., Magnani, L., Barosi, G.: An epistemological framework for medical knowledge-based systems. IEEE Trans. Syst. Man Cybern. **22**, 1361–1375 (1992)

Rich, B.A.: Defining and delineating a duty to prognosticate. Theor. Med. Bioeth. **22**(3), 177–192 (2001)

Rich, B.A.: Prognostication in clinical medicine: prophecy or professional responsibility? J. Leg. Med. **23**(3), 297–358 (2002)

Risjord, M.: Nursing Knowledge: Science, Practice, and Philosophy. Wiley-Blackwell, Oxford (2011)

Rizzi, D.A.: Medical prognosis—some fundamentals. Theoret. Med. **14**(4), 365–375 (1993)

Sadegh-Zadeh, K.: Handbook of Analytic Philosophy of Medicine. Springer, Dordrecht (2012)

Salmon, W.C.: Statistical explanation. In: Colodny, R.G. (ed.) The Nature and Function of Scientific Theories, pp. 173–231. Reidel, Dordrecht, Holland (1970)

Smith, A.K., White, D.B., Arnold, R.M.: Uncertainty: the other side of prognosis. N. Engl. J. Med. **368**(26), 2448–2450 (2013)

Stanley, D.E., Campos, D.G.: The logic of medical diagnosis. Perspect. Biol. Med. **56**(2), 300–315 (2013)

Stanley, D.E., Campos, D.G.: Selecting clinical diagnoses: logical strategies informed by experience. J. Eval. Clin. Pract. **22**(4), 588–597 (2016)

Thagard, P.: Conceptual Revolutions. Princeton University Press, Princeton (1992)

Thagard, P.: Abductive inference: from philosophical analysis to neural mechanisms. In: Feeney, A., Heit, E. (eds.) Inductive Reasoning: Cognitive, Mathematical, and Neuroscientific Approaches, pp. 226–247. Cambridge University Press, Cambridge (2006)

Thorne, S., Sawatzky, R.: Particularizing the general: sustaining theoretical integrity in the context of an evidence-based practice agenda. Adv. Nurs. Sci. **37**(1), 5–18 (2014)

Tonelli, M.R.: In defense of expert opinion. Acad. Med. **74**(11), 1187–1192 (1999)

Upshur, R.: Certainty, probability and abduction: why we should look to CS Peirce rather than Gödel for a theory of clinical reasoning. J. Eval. Clin. Pract. **3**(3), 201–206 (1997)

Walton, D.: Abductive Reasoning. University of Alabama Press, Tuscaloosa (2004)

Wiesemann, C.: The significance of prognosis for a theory of medical practice. Theor. Med. Bioeth. **19**(3), 253–261 (1998)

Woods, J.: Errors of Reasoning. Naturalizing the Logic of Inference. College Publications, London (2013)

Chapter 5
Prognosis in the Face of Uncertainty

5.1 Introduction

Reasoning in medicine requires the critical use of a clinical methodology whose validity and limits must be evaluated. Methodological questions are at the heart of the research in clinical reasoning: they concern, on the one hand, a more objective approach to medicine based on biomedical evidence and explanations in which signs convey clinical information; and, on the other, a person-centred medicine in which clinical signs have a meaning also within the individual's human experience.

In general, evidence in medicine does not have the same intuitive features as in other research fields. Evidence Based Medicine (EBM), for instance, erroneously assumes that the nature of scientific evidence in medicine has in recent decades changed profoundly thanks to the methodological development of clinical research, in particular for what concerns the collection of clinical information and the tools for their analysis. EBM in its most orthodox formulation claims to offer the clinician "certainties" or "truths", simply by differentiating between the most and the least reliable data, or between "scientific" and "less scientific" facts. And, to do this, EBM suffices to consider as evidence only the results obtained through the most rigorous methodology, i.e. randomized controlled trials (RCTs). Such an epistemological attitude is too optimistic (resembling certain perspectives of the first logical positivism) because it considers the execution of rigorous experiments as a necessary and sufficient condition to know reality. Also, this is a very simplified view of medical epistemology, which does not take into account the complexity of medical research (see for example Clarke et al. 2014; Djulbegovic et al. 2009; Cartwright 2007).

In recent years the methodological limitations of this approach have emerged even more clearly following the so-called "reproducibility crisis" (Ioannidis 2005). The

D. Chiffi, *Clinical Reasoning: Knowledge, Uncertainty, and Values in Health Care,* Studies in Applied Philosophy, Epistemology and Rational Ethics 58, https://doi.org/10.1007/978-3-030-59094-9_5

exponential increase in scientific publications and their sensationalist nature (especially in the biomedical field) have led many researchers to doubt and to question much of scientific production. The numerous attempts to replicate scientific studies published in the most prestigious international journals have given alarming results: only a small percentage has proved to be reproducible (Baker 2015; Morrison 2014). Epidemiological research is not an exception. Several studies have highlighted the numerous methodological biases that afflict clinical trials, one of the most frequent of which is the inadequate number of samples used. Among others, the epidemiologist John Ioannidis has dealt with this problem. One of his most well-known works, in fact, concerns the empirical evaluation of the so-called "very large effects" (VLE) of therapeutic interventions[1] (Ioannidis 2005). The epidemiologists involved in this paper identified all the studies that demonstrated the existence of VLE in the Cochrane Database of Systematic Reviews; then, they searched the literature for further trials that could confirm or deny them. The result was quite disconcerting: all the results initially identified as VLE became much smaller or even disappeared in later studies. After an in-depth analysis, it was found that the studies showing VLEs were all under-powered, i.e. the sample size used was very small. In a clinical trial without an adequate sample, it is very difficult to distinguish the observation of a random fluctuation from a real effect (Andreoletti and Teira 2016). In these cases, it is not possible to observe the same effect again simply because there is none. This means that the evidence that EBM wants to rely on in order to offer certainties to the doctor appears to be anything but reliable. As we have seen, *prima facie* the EBM epistemology fails in reducing the complexity of medical science. And yet, recognizing the limits of epidemiological evidence does not automatically mean to deny its epistemic value, which should instead be reaffirmed in a context in which the complexity of medicine is managed through tools such as critical reasoning and logic. In other terms, doubt and uncertainty, and not certainty, should be the foundation of contemporary medical epistemology (Djulbegovic 2007). As pointed out by Eddy (1984, p. 75):

> Uncertainty creeps into medical practice through every pore. Whether a physician is defining a disease, making a diagnosis, selecting a procedure, observing outcomes, assessing probabilities, assigning preferences, or putting it all together, he is walking on a very slippery terrain. It is difficult for nonphysicians, and for many physicians, to appreciate how complex these tasks are, how poorly we understand them, and how easy it is for honest people to come to different conclusions.

Starting from recent criticism toward medical evidence, I will try to understand its potential theoretical and clinical implications with respect to the nature of prognosis (Sect. 5.2). Moreover, I will investigate the pragmatic and illocutionary aspects of different forms of linguistic acts and judgments (Austin 1962; Searle 1969) that are involved in clinical practice and are key features of clinical reasoning and communication. In Sect. 5.3, I will then explore the role of uncertainty in connection with

---

[1]In small sample settings, statistical power analysis that usually relies on statistical significance may face methodological limitations. Specific design calculations have been recently suggested (Gelman and Carlin 2014).

general and particular clinical judgments, and its relation with the general epidemi-ological evidence, in particular for the formulation of diagnostic judgments. In Sect. 5.4, I will focus on the explication, structure and limits of (the concept of) prognosis and how prognostic judgments are formulated and justified. Section 5.5 concludes the chapter.

5.2 Evidence and Clinical Reasoning

In the last decades, philosophers of science have been investigating and criticizing the concept of evidence in medicine and have put the limits of EBM epistemology into discussion. There is a wide scholarly consensus that evidence from RCTs is insufficient to establish a causal link between an intervention and its effect. As far as interventions are concerned, medical scientists need to possess mechanistic knowl-edge of how the intervention brings about its effect. This is precisely why medical decisions that are made based on RCTs results alone are prone to errors[2]: physicians should consider obtaining evidence from other sources as well. Recent evidence from meta-research is also seriously questioning the validity of RCTs, since several biases actually distort the results of such studies. Some philosophers and (meta-)scientists have suggested that we lower our degree of belief in medical interventions. For example, Stegenga (2018) has defended the idea of "medical nihilism", opting for a more realistic understanding of what medical practice can and cannot achieve. Fuller (2018) has also recently argued for updating (lowering) our confidence in medical claims based on meta-research evidence, in order to avoid being irrational. On his part, the leading meta-research scholar Ioannidis (2008) advocates, more pragmati-cally, for a "rational down-adjustment of effect sizes" usually found in the medical literature.

So far, philosophical analysis of medical practice has focused mostly on inter-ventions, while other important areas of medicine, such as diagnosis and to a greater extent prognosis, have not gained much attention. Diagnostic and prognostic judg-ments require a different reasoning process—and a different type of evidence—than interventions. When patients receive a diagnosis of a disease, they are not just inter-ested in finding out about their recovery, but also want to know what will happen to them in terms of the natural course of the disease and quality of life. In short, they care about *their own prognosis*. For example, patients who have been diagnosed with cancer want to know if they will die, if something painful will happen to them, and what kind of life they can lead following the diagnosis. This sort of information is not just interesting per se, but has profound impact on the patient's decisions about treatment. Patients can decide to undergo "harmful" treatments if their conditions have a very bad course, or forget about having treatment if the disease does not have much impact on their quality of life.

---

[2]However, also mechanistic knowledge may be fallacious or at least not optimal when clinical phenomena assume a systemic structure.

Prognosis relates to the anticipated results of a disease or situation and the likelihood of its occurrence. Further expanding the definition, prognosis involves the effect of a disease or situation over time and the projected likelihood of regeneration or continuing related morbidity, with a given a set of variables called prognostic factors or indices of prognosis (see e.g. Moons et al. 2009). Prognostic factors can help clinicians predict which patients are more or less likely to experience a given outcome. For example, we can predict death events or disability at 5 years in stroke survivals: patients who have moderate hemiparesis at baseline are 3 times more likely to die or be disabled at 5 years, whereas those with severe hemiparesis are over 4 times more likely to die or be disabled (Fineout-Overholt and Mazurek Melnyk 2004).

A rough search on the PubMed database for papers that use the terms "prognostic factor" in the title and abstract is enough to see how prognostic research has grown significantly in the last decade. Prognostic research shows to be a fundamental sort of inquiry within the emerging paradigm of "personalized medicine" or "precision medicine". Nowadays, these two terms are ubiquitous in medical journals, popular science, social networks, and so forth. Even multinational tech companies, such as Google, Apple, Amazon, etc. are investing in personalized healthcare research. There is indeed unanimous consensus among all the relevant stakeholders that precision medicine will be the next big revolution in healthcare. In principle, personalized or precision medicine is not confined to the effectiveness of treatments or preventive strategies, but rather "addresses how to use an individual's prognostic information to make personally tailored choices about the best-suited treatment or preventive management" (Moons et al. 2018). This is why studies on prognostic and predictive factors (markers) and models have become abundant in the medical literature. As of today, for instance, we can observe growing popularity of studies that investigate the staging of cancers to predict the progression of the disease and the survival rates, as well as of studies that analyse genetic markers to predict individual response to treatments. But, as economists have taught us, high demand means that supply increases. Although prognostic research is being progressively rewarded publication-wise, its growth is dismally taking place more in terms of quantity than of quality.

Recently, an increasing body of empirical evidence has highlighted the severe limitations of prognostic research. For instance, Riley et al. (2019) have shown in what way prognostic studies can often be poorly designed. Altman et al. (1994) highlighted severe flaws in the analysis of the data, and McShane et al. (2006) noticed that results are being poorly reported, to say the least. All in all, after an initial period of excitement, the community is given less and less credit to prognostic studies. Fishing for significant correlations is now a notorious attitude, especially in some disease areas. Poorly designed prognostic research has been wryly labelled as a "playground" for researchers, or even "what's in the fridge approach" (see Riley et al. 2019). Apparently, the famous "correlation is not causation", which has been repeated by everyone over the years as a mantra, did not have any effect at all.

Medical researchers and institutions, like the Cochrane Collaboration, are actively working to standardize and improve prognostic research to facilitate medical decision making. Still, as of today, it is evident that the vast majority of prognostic studies are not fully reliable.

The problem of reasoning under uncertainty in the context of personalized medicine has been recently discussed by Walker et al. (2019). While in basic science novel methods of gaining evidence—such as iPSc (induced Pluripotent Stem Cells)— are being generated (Boniolo 2016), such shortcuts are still far from being achieved in a clinical setting (Andreoletti 2018). Therefore, a more detailed and philosophical analysis of prognostic judgments might be helpful.

5.3 General and Particular Medical Assertions

It is well-known that any prognosis requires a diagnosis. In this section, I am going to explore the role of different levels of medical judgments and assertions. More specifically, I focus on the speech acts involved in diagnostic and prognostic judgments and on their connection with epidemiological evidence. An internal judgment, in fact, can be externally expressed with different speech acts in clinical communication. The issue of epidemiological evidence obviously plays an important role not only in supporting the critical judgment on the patient's health conditions, but also in supporting the diagnostic and prognostic judgment and the choice of therapy. On the one hand, a specific diagnosis is inevitably linked to the medical knowledge and epidemiological evidence available in a given historical period: if the epidemiological evidence is conflicting or unreliable, then even the diagnostic judgment based on such evidence could be incorrect. On the other hand, usually clinicians do not base their judgment simply on epidemiological evidence but attempt to understand how and to what extent the evidence from epidemiological studies can inform their judgment once signs, symptoms and any other information on the patient's state of heath are taken into account (Thorne and Sawatzky 2014). Thus, there seems to be, at least *prima facie*, a continuous and mutual interplay between what Federspil and Vettor (2001) call "general medical assertions" and what we might call, using similar terminology, "particular medical assertions".[3] Generally, an assertion is an illocutionary act that must satisfy certain standards of acceptability in order to be considered justified.[4] In this sense, different levels of acceptability can be thought to justifiably assert a proposition. For example, an assertion can be considered justified if it is true, if it is known, if there is evidence, or if it is reasonable to believe it is true. Though, medical assertions seem to have a specific nature. Clinicians, in fact, may deem an assertion justified not only by its truth or knowledge value, but also by the possibility of proving or attempting to corroborate a proposition (given the knowledge and medical evidence available). This last point of view, in particular, is usually accepted in EBM.

In EBM, the notion of evidence is connected with the notion of proof, meaning that a general medical assertion requires proof of its content to be justified. But, as we have seen, the notion of justification refers (at least implicitly) to some notion of

---

[3] On the connection between the speech act of assertion and diagnostic judgment, see Schulz (2006).
[4] For a pragmatic logic for assertions and other speech acts, see Carrara et al. (2017).

norm or threshold of evidence acceptance. General medical assertions seem to have the following structure: given a proposition that expresses a medical thesis, we try to understand if the degree of evidence achieved through epidemiological studies, meta-analyses and systematic reviews of the literature allows us to be confident in the thesis so as to assert it in a justified manner. The following fundamental issues emerge, therefore, when analysing general medical assertions according to the EBM:

1. as noted by Federspil and Vettor (2001), the idea of evidence held by EBM does not take into due consideration that the available medical evidence allows us to confer different degrees of credibility to our medical theses with regard to the *different theoretical frameworks of reference*. Forms of evidence that seem to justify a medical assertion could be unjustified in a different theoretical framework or for different clinical purposes.[5]
2. like any empirical knowledge, even medical assertions can never be conclusively proven and are always subject to a risk of error.
3. the choice of the evidentiary thresholds to consider an assertion as justified is conventionally established (in particular the thresholds for false positives and false negatives) but may vary based on epistemic and non-epistemic considerations (Hempel 1965).

The justification of particular medical assertions is perhaps an even more complex issue. Suffice it to recall that the data of a reference population or the evidence of clinical trials can in some cases show no traces of a clinical judgment referring to a single patient. Often, trials do not include patients with comorbidity, a very common situation with elderly patients. Even if the evidence at the general population level is, at least in principle, clinically relevant for the formulation of a particular clinical assertion, it may be difficult to isolate the factors of clinical relevance that allow us to select a reference partition of a single patient's particular pathological condition (Giaretta and Chiffi 2018). Finally, particular medical assertions are difficult to justify either because a disease can show a high individual variability, or because the experimental conditions do not reflect those commonly encountered in clinical practice. Nonetheless, even if fallible, diagnosis can be viewed as a particular medical assertion, since it is always about a specific patient in a precise time. The uncertainty permeating a diagnosis is usually not severe and can be statistically assessed; on the contrary, the uncertainty permeating prognostic judgments is more significant, as we will see in the next section.

5.4 Prognostic Judgment: Structure and Uncertainty

There are many reasons behind the fact that prognosis has received so far much less clinical and philosophical interest than diagnosis, the most important being the deep

---

[5]However, some exceptions to this are also contemplated within EBM as we will see in the case of the best evidence required for prognostication.

uncertainty of the future permeating prognostic judgment. As we have seen, the aim of prognostics is to judge: (i) the duration of a specific future stage of a disease in a given patient, (ii) the probability of a patient recovering from a disease, or (iii) the chances of a patient's survival (Rizzi 1993). All these aims of prognosis are intimately connected with other stages of clinical reasoning such as the ascertainment of a diagnosis and the choice of therapy. This means that a prognosis inevitably requires a diagnosis, and that the selection of the proper therapy for a patient is based on different prognostic scenarios.

The logical structure of prognosis is not always fully explicated. A clear explication of a notion, instead, may prevent forms of ambiguity that can negatively affect clinical reasoning and medical decisions. One interesting explication[6] of prognosis is provided by Sadegh-Zadeh (2012), who defines a prognosis (π) as:

$$\pi = (p, D, KB \cup M) \tag{5.1}$$

where p indicates a specific patient, D stands for patient's data, KB is the knowledge base used to substantiate the clinician's formulation of the prognosis, and M is the method of reasoning and argumentation adopted for the prognosis. This explication is valuable, but I think there is still room to clarify some of its components and possibly extend it.

I hold that KB is a crucial ingredient of this explication and includes many different aspects such as (i) the awareness of epidemiological data (ED) with reference to specific populations of patients; (ii) the level of expertise (E) of the clinician in dealing with similar patients; (iii) the connection (C) (if meaningful) between epidemiological (population) data and the development of the patient's disease.

Based on this, we can postulate that

$$KB = (ED, E, C). \tag{5.2}$$

As previously mentioned, the connection C may be particularly problematic since it consists in (i) finding a meaningful reference class in population studies and (ii) attempting to 'particularize' the relevant clinical factors of that class to a specific patient (see Chiffi and Pietarinen 2019; Fuller and Flores 2015). What is often lacking is some guidance to the use of a clinician's judgment in shaping the variety of sources of information to a specific case. On the one hand, finding a relevant population class from the trial can sometimes be hopeless since experimental conditions—as we have seen—can hardly be replicated in clinical practice; on the other hand, given the

---

[6]I think that it may be useful to recall here again what an explication is. An explication is intended to capture the core meaning of a notion, ruling out the less relevant part of it. In other terms, an explication is a procedure of conceptual clarification of a vague concept, the *explicandum*, with a precise concept, the *explicatum*, so that the *explicatum* must be: (i) similar to the explicandum; (ii) more exact and informative than the *explicandum*; (iii) simple in order to be easily formalized; and finally (iv) connected by means of the explication with a rigorous system of scientific concepts (Carnap 1950). A different sense of explication is the Kantian one for which explication does not require condition (iii), i.e. the condition of formalization. See Boniolo (2003).

intricacy of individual variability, the criteria for the resemblance of the patient with the population may not be fully accurate. A common epidemiological and clinical view in order to calibrate function C deals with "accepting that results of randomized trials apply to wide population unless there is a compelling reason to believe the results would differ substantially as a function of particular characteristics of those patients" (Post et al. 2013, pp. 641–642; see also Dans et al. 1998). As observed by Fuller (2019), this can be viewed as a sort of "presumption of generalizability" that resembles the *argumentum ad ignorantiam* in argumentation theory, which has the following form: it is not known (proved) that a proposition A is true (false), therefore A is false (true) (Woods and Walton 1978). Even if this form of reasoning is not always fallacious, it remains particularly problematic when the specific knowledge base is far from being complete and reliable. This is almost always the case for medical evidence and knowledge, since "negative arguments depend on the completeness of the negated paradigm. In medicine or history, such a paradigm can be hardly considered as complete, and therefore reasoning from ignorance can only provide a certain degree of probability" (Macagno and Walton 2011, p. 99; see also Walton 1996). This means that the issue of establishing sound methodological and clinical rules in order to select the proper connection between epidemiological and clinical evidence, is difficult and may represent the hallmark of sound clinical reasoning.

Let us consider again the proposed explication of prognosis. At any rate, the explication π of prognosis is in a strict sense the propositional content (intended as the final result) of an *act* of prognostication. The act of prognostication is a *verdictive* illocutionary act, in which a specific judgment or verdict is claimed and justified even in the presence of uncertainty. Because of the illocutionary act of prognosis, many perlocutionary effects may follow as is, in fact, the case for a patient receiving a prognosis. Austin classically pointed out that

> verdictives, are typified by the giving of a verdict, as the name implies, by a jury, arbitrator, or umpire. But they need not be final; they may be, for example, an estimate, reckoning, or appraisal. It is essentially giving a finding as to something-fact, or value which is for different reasons hard to be certain about. (Austin 1962, p. 151)

To which the author adds:

> Verdictives consist in the delivering of a finding, official or unofficial, upon evidence or reasons as to value or fact, so far as these are distinguishable. (Austin 1962, p. 152)

Verdictive acts, thus, occur under a veil of uncertainty, while, for instance, the act of assertion requires something similar to conclusive evidence for its justification. In the light of these considerations and the standard pragmatic distinction between the speech act and the (propositional) content, if we are to indicate the illocutionary act of prognostication by P, the general form of an act of prognostication is the following:

$$P(\pi) \tag{5.3}$$

which is equivalent, in virtue of (5.1) to

$$P(p, D, KB \cup M) \tag{5.4}$$

and by (5.2), we have that (5.4) is equivalent to

$$P(p, D, ((ED, E, C) \cup M)). \tag{5.5}$$

The formula in (5.5) indicates the general form of a prognostic judgment expressed by means of an illocutionary and verdictive act, whose propositional content delivers information regarding: the patient, the health data of the patient, the knowledge base of the clinician consisting in epidemiological evidence, professional expertise, and the relation between epidemiological and clinical evidence once a clinical reasoning method is used. Since prognostics is usually permeated by uncertainty, the methods of clinical reasoning are standardly based on a probabilistic assessments; however, in case of severe forms of uncertainty, difficult to be handled by probabilities, also abductive or 'retroductive' forms of reasoning may have something to say (Pietarinen and Bellucci 2014). In fact, in the case in which not all the ingredients of a prognosis are fully recognized and listed, we can talk of an incomplete or elliptic prognosis.

The explication (5.5) can be used to understand disagreement among clinicians about prognostication, especially with regard to the development of a disease in the very same patient. Forms of disagreement may arise from various factors such as clinical and epidemiological considerations, the similarity between the health conditions of a patient and a relevant reference class, the different forms of reasoning used in formulating the prognostic judgments, and so forth.

As noticed before, for any illocutionary act, there should be some justification conditions supporting the felicity of the execution of that act. In the case of prognostication, we want the prognosis to be about a future event. The idea here is that pathophysiological considerations and epidemiological evidence should contribute to assessing a future stage of the disease in a specific patient. Yet, pathophysiological considerations, or more in general causal considerations, are not always required for a prognosis, since statistical associations may provide the proper ground to formulate it (Stovitz and Shrier 2019).

Choosing which form of evidence is better to use for prognostication is rather difficult. EBM practitioners hold that RCTs are considered inappropriate when the study is looking at the prognosis of a disease. We can read, for instance, that:

a special type of cohort study may also be used to determine the prognosis of a disease (i.e. what is likely to happen to someone who has it). A group of people who have all been diagnosed as having an early stage of the disease or a positive screening test [...] is assembled (the inception cohort) and followed up on repeated occasions to see the incidence (new cases per year) and time course of different outcomes. (Greenhalgh 2010, p. 38)

The failure to select a proper inception cohort may result in unpredictable effects and fatal flow on prognostic studies (Ales and Charlson 1987). As pointed out by Mebius et al. (2016) there seems to exist 'an apparent contradiction' between *best evidence in general*, which is usually assumed in EBM to come from RCTs (and meta-analyses of their findings), and the *best evidence for prognostic purposes*, which comes from inception cohorts, defined as "a group of individuals identified and assembled for subsequent study at an early and uniform point in the course of the specified health condition" (Porta 2014). This is a nice example of how the goodness of evidence can change based on its use and on the different theoretical frameworks it is grounded on. However, it is a known fact that observational studies are never free of bias, which is even more relevant for prognostic studies, often flawed with poor methodological standards (Lim and Feldman 2013). Not by chance, some epidemiologists pointed out that, whenever clinicians select prognostic studies to inform their practice and happen to encounter a study for which no inception cohort was assembled, they should just move on to the next article (Clinical Epidemiological Round, Canadian Medical Association 1981). For instance, if only current patients would be studied for prognosis—being the ones who had the most severe disease already died—then the observed outcomes would be overly optimistic.

A prognosis is almost always more uncertain than a diagnosis (Chiffi and Zanotti 2017), and the reliability of available prognostic tools remains limited (Riley et al. 2013). In fact, a prognosis can be perfectly rational, but still wrong because of the irreducible uncertainty permeating the act of prognostication. This is due to the fact that many aspects of the future are intrinsically unknown and difficult to be probabilistically evaluated. On this point, von Mises (1966) considered necessary to distinguish between, on the one side, the *class probability*, in which the frequency of a certain homogeneous class is known, but the behaviour of the individual outcomes of the class cannot be identified; and on the other side, the *case probability*, typical of the disciplines that are shaped by teleological aspects, which deals with unique events that cannot be grouped into larger classes. Likewise, the evolution of a disease in a specific patient can be inherently unpredictable.[7] Also, (particular) clinical prognostic judgments have to deal with lifestyles, compliance with therapy, ideas, values and contingencies of patients. As a way of example, some years ago a friend of mine who was a talented professor of philosophical logic consciously decided not to receive chemotherapeutic treatments to cure his cancer, preferring to undergo awake brain surgery. His motivation was that he did not want to lose his cognitive capacities (something fundamental for a logician), even if life expectancy would have decreased dramatically. Unfortunately, one year after receiving his cancer diagnosis he passed away, leaving a permanent mark on many people both in and outside academia. This is a clear example of both the dramatic role of the patient's views about the future in changing the prognosis, and of all the limits in explicating the very concept of prognosis. However, the proposed explication of prognostic judgment may help us understand some sources of clinical uncertainty. For instance, it may be the case that: (i) diseases—as we have seen—may develop in unpredictable ways; (ii) for some diseases the behaviour, lifestyles, values, and therapeutic patients' preferences may affect the reliability of the prognosis; (iii) the clinical framework assigned to a patient is scarcely known or even incorrect; (iv) the epidemiological and medical knowledge

---

[7]The question of fundamental uncertainty that can be hardly analysed from a probabilistic point of view is also investigated by Keynes (1948) and the neo-Keynesian school.

base used by the clinician to substantiate the prognostic judgment is incomplete or not updated; (v) the reasoning and argumentative methods are fallacious.

At any rate, (5.5) does not claim to be an exhaustive definition of the act of prognosis, but rather an explication collecting the main relevant ingredients of a prognosis that may rule out some specific aspects. A patient's values and choices may induce clinicians to formulate an alternative prognosis and to imagine an alternative future course of events, that is better aligned with the patient's decisions, just as long as such decisions are well substantiated, sound and informed. And, even though the merits of an objective explication of the act of prognosis are undeniable, we cannot but recognise that it falls short in providing a patient-centred approach to prognostication able to include the patient's values and decisions and the way he/she conceives the uncertainty of the future. This fact highlights, once again, how the practice of medicine is an art in which both the patient and the doctor have much to say. The proposed pragmatic analysis attempted to reveal the merit of a linguistic and argumentative approach to prognostication and thus pave the way to a critical reflection on such a fundamental step in clinical reasoning.

5.5 Conclusion

Clinical reasoning and communication show a pragmatic and illocutionary structure. In this chapter, I have clarified the role and the justification conditions of clinical judgments in dealing with fundamental forms of uncertainty in future scenarios. Current epidemiological evidence can hardly be replicated, inducing oftentimes the physician to refine the methodology of clinical reasoning in order to come up with accurate judgments. Clinical judgments may be externally communicated by means of different illocutionary acts. I have identified general medical assertions, in which clinical claims are not associated to a single patient but remain at population level, and particular medical assertions, which are instead patient's specific (see, also Giaretta and Federspil 1998). Then, I focused on prognostic judgment and pointed out that a prognosis is usually communicated as a form of verdictive speech act, which often occurs under fundamental uncertainty and which includes to claim something regarding a future clinical event. In the light of this, I have extended and integrated Sadegh-Zadeh's explication of prognosis, by analysing the nature of the knowledge base used by clinicians and by showing validity and limits of the proposed explication. The difficulties of shaping the prognostic judgment based on epidemiological data and clinical signs and symptoms have been underlined. Such connection is usually warranted in EBM by means of the "presumption of generalizability" of the findings of RCTs, which is a form of *argument ad ignorantiam*. This argument may be fallacious in those fields that are permeated by fundamental uncertainty such as clinical reasoning. Finally, I have critically discussed the fact that the main reason behind the failure of an objective explication of the act of prognosis seems to rely on the subjective features associated with patient's values, decisions and behaviours.

Prognosis is, indeed, uncertain inasmuch as our single lives are uncertain. Nevertheless, clinical reasoning may help us to mitigate and better understand such uncertainty and to soundly communicate it.

References

Ales, K.L., Charlson, M.E.: In search of the true inception cohort. J. Chron. Dis. **40**(9), 881–885 (1987)

Altman, D.G., Lausen, B., Sauerbrei, W., Schumacher, M.: Dangers of using "optimal" cutpoints in the evaluation of prognostic factors. JNCI J. Natl. Cancer Inst. **86**(11), 829–835 (1994)

Andreoletti, M.: More than one way to measure? A casuistic approach to cancer clinical trials. Perspect. Biol. Med. **61**(2), 174–190 (2018)

Andreoletti, M., Teira, D.: Statistical evidence and the reliability of medical research. In: Solomon, M., Jeremy, J.R., Simon, Kincaid, H. (eds.) The Routledge Companion to Philosophy of Medicine, pp. 232–241. Routledge, London (2016)

Austin, J.L.: How to Do Things with Words. Oxford University Press, Oxford (1962)

Baker, M.: Over half of psychology studies fail reproducibility test. Nat. News (2015). https://doi.org/10.1038/nature.2015.18248

Boniolo, G.: Kant's explication and Carnap's explication: the *redde rationem*. Int. Philos. Q. **43**(3), 289–298 (2003)

Boniolo, G.: Molecular medicine: the clinical method enters the lab. In: Boniolo, G., Nathan, M.J. (eds.) Philosophy of Molecular Medicine, pp. 23–42. Routledge, London (2016)

Carnap, R.: Logical Foundations of Probability. University of Chicago Press, Chicago (1950)

Carrara, M., Chiffi, D., De Florio, C.: Assertions and hypotheses: a logical framework for their oppositions relations. Logic J. IGPL **25**(2), 131–144 (2017)

Cartwright, N.: Are RCTs the gold standard? BioSocieties **2**(1), 11–20 (2007)

Chiffi, D., Pietarinen, A.V.: Clinical equipoise and moral leeway: an epistemological stance. Topoi **38**(2), 447–456 (2019)

Chiffi, D., Zanotti, R.: Fear of knowledge: clinical hypotheses in diagnostic and prognostic reasoning. J. Eval. Clin. Pract. **23**(5), 928–934 (2017)

Clarke, B., Gillies, D., Illari, P., Russo, F., Williamson, J.: Mechanisms and the evidence hierarchy. Topoi **33**(2), 339–360 (2014)

Clinical Epidemiological Round (Canadian Medical Association): How to read clinical journals: III. To learn the clinical course and prognosis of disease. CMAJ **124**(7), 869–872 (1981)

Dans, A.L., Dans, L.F., Guyatt, G.H., Richardson, S.: Evidence-based medicine working group: users' guides to the medical literature: XIV. How to decide on the applicability of clinical trial results to your patient. JAMA **279**(7), 545–549 (1998)

Djulbegovic, B.: Articulating and responding to uncertainties in clinical research. J. Med. Philos. **32**(2), 79–98 (2007)

Djulbegovic, B., Guyatt, G.H., Ashcroft, R.E.: Epistemologic inquiries in evidence-based medicine. Cancer Control **16**(2), 158–168 (2009)

Eddy, D.M.: Variations in physician practice: the role of uncertainty. Health Aff. **3**(2), 74–89 (1984)

Federspil, G., Vettor, R.: La "evidence-based medicine": una riflessione critica sul concetto di evidenza in medicina. Ital. Heart J. **2**(6 Suppl), 614–623 (2001)

Fineout-Overholt, E., Mazurek Melnyk, B.: Evaluation of studies of prognosis. Evid.-Based Nurs. **7**(1), 4–8 (2004)

Fuller, J.: Meta-research evidence for evaluating therapies. Philos. Sci. **85**(5), 767–780 (2018)

Fuller, J.: The myth and fallacy of simple extrapolation in medicine. Synthese (2019). https://doi.org/10.1007/s11229-019-02255-0

Fuller, J., Flores, L.J.: The risk GP model: the standard model of prediction in medicine. Stud. Hist. Philos. Sci. Part C Stud. Hist. Philos. Biol. Biomed. Sci. **54**, 49–61 (2015)

Gelman, A., Carlin, J.: Beyond power calculations: assessing type S (sign) and type M (magnitude) errors. Perspect. Psychol. Sci. **9**(6), 641–651 (2014)

Giaretta, P., Federspil, G.: Il procedimento clinico. Analisi logica di un caso. Piccin, Padova (1998)

Giaretta, P., Chiffi, D.: Varieties of probability in clinical diagnosis. Acta Balt. Hist. Philos. Sci. **6**(1), 5–27 (2018)

Greenhalgh, T.: How to Read a Paper: The Basics of Evidence-Based Medicine. Wiley, Chichester, West Sussex (2010)

Hempel, C.G.: Science and human values. In: Aspects of Scientific Explanation and Other Essays in the Philosophy of Science, pp. 81–96. The Free Press, New York (1965)

Ioannidis, J.P.: Why most published research findings are false. PLoS Med. **2**(8), e124 (2005)

Ioannidis, J.P.: Why most discovered true associations are inflated. Epidemiology **19**(5), 640–648 (2008)

Keynes, J.M.: A Treatise on Probability. Macmillan, London (1948)

Lim, L.S.H., Feldman, B.M.: The risky business of studying prognosis. J. Rheumatol. **40**(1), 9–15 (2013)

Macagno, F., Walton, D.: Reasoning from paradigms and negative evidence. Pragmat. Cogn. **19**(1), 92–116 (2011)

McShane, L.M., Altman, D.G., Sauerbrei, W., Taube, S.E., Gion, M., Clark, G.M.: REporting recommendations for tumor MARKer prognostic studies (REMARK). Breast Cancer Res. Treat. **100**(2), 229–235 (2006)

Mebius, A., Kennedy, A.G., Howick, J.: Research gaps in the philosophy of evidence-based medicine. Philos. Compass **11**(11), 757–771 (2016)

Mises, L.: Human Action, a Treatise on Economics. Henry Regnery, Chicago (1966)

Moons, K.G.M., Royston, P., Vergouwe, Y., Grobbee, D.E., Altman, D.G.: Prognosis and prognostic research: what, why, and how? BMJ **338**, b375 (2009)

Moons, K.G.M., Hooft, L., Williams, K., Hayden, J.A., Damen, J.A.A.G., Riley, R.D.: Implementing systematic reviews of prognosis studies in Cochrane. Cochrane Database Syst. Rev. **10** (2018). Art. No.: ED000129. https://doi.org/10.1002/14651858.ED000129

Morrison, S.J.: Reproducibility project: cancer biology: time to do something about reproducibility. Elife **3**, e03981 (2014)

Pietarinen, A.V., Bellucci, F.: New light on Peirce's conceptions of retroduction, deduction, and scientific reasoning. Int. Stud. Philos. Sci. **28**(4), 353–373 (2014)

Porta, M.: A Dictionary of Epidemiology, 6th edn. Oxford University Press, New York (2014)

Post, P.N., de Beer, H., Guyatt, G.H.: How to generalize efficacy results of randomized trials: recommendations based on a systematic review of possible approaches. J. Eval. Clin. Pract. **19**(4), 638–643 (2013)

Riley, R.D., Hayden, J.A., Steyerberg, E.W., Moons, K.G.M., Abrams, K., Kyzas, P.A., Hemingway, H.: Prognosis research strategy (PROGRESS) 2: prognostic factor research. PLoS Med. **10**(2), e1001380 (2013)

Riley, R.D., van der Windt, D., Croft, P., Moons, K.G. (eds.): Prognosis Research in Healthcare: Concepts, Methods, and Impact. Oxford University Press, Oxford (2019)

Rizzi, D.A.: Medical prognosis—some fundamentals. Theor. Med. Bioeth. **14**(4), 365–375 (1993)

Sadegh-Zadeh, K.: Handbook of Analytic Philosophy of Medicine. Springer, Dordrecht (2012)

Schulz, P.J.: The communication of diagnostic information by doctors to patients in the consultation. In: Kalitzkus, V., Twohig, P.L. (eds.) Bordering Biomedicine, pp. 103–118. Rodopi, Amsterdam, New York (2006)

Searle, J.R.: Speech Acts: An Essay in the Philosophy of Language. Cambridge University Press, Cambridge (1969)

Stegenga, J.: Medical Nihilism. Oxford University Press, Oxford (2018)

Stovitz, S.D., Shrier, I.: Causal inference for clinicians. BMJ Evid.-Based Med. BMJ EBM (2019)

Thorne, S., Sawatzky, R.: Particularizing the general: sustaining theoretical integrity in the context of an evidence-based practice agenda. Adv. Nurs. Sci. **37**(1), 5–18 (2014)

Walker, M.J., Bourke, J., Hutchison, K.: Evidence for personalised medicine: mechanisms, correlation, and new kinds of black box. Theor. Med. Bioeth. **40**(2), 103–121 (2019)

Walton, D.: Arguments from Ignorance. Pennsylvania State University Press, University Park, PA (1996)

Woods, J., Walton, D.: The fallacy of 'ad ignorantiam.' Dialectica **32**(2), 87–99 (1978)

Part II
Philosophy of Clinical Reasoning, Research and Practice

Chapter 6
On Clinical Possibility

6.1 Introduction

One category of concepts, which has been extensively analysed in logic and philosophy and which may contribute to critical reflection on clinical knowledge, diagnoses and interventions, concerns modal notions. Modalities are defined as "ways in which something can exist or occur or be presented, or stand" (Proudfoot and Lacey 2009, p. 258). Despite the common use of modal concepts in clinical reasoning, analysis of their role in clinical contexts is almost absent in the literature.[1] Among the most widely recognized kinds of modality, we find *alethic modalities*, which concern the modes of presenting the concept of truth; *epistemic modalities*, which regard the agents' knowledge; and *deontic modalities*, which deal with situations related to a certain system of values and laws.[2] Likewise, possibility, which is one of the most commonly used concepts of modality, includes various kinds: logical possibility, for instance, regards a state of things that does not violate any logical law, whereas physical possibility regards a state of things that do not contradict physical laws. Clearly, physical possibility entails the logical one, but not vice versa, and the same also holds true for other kinds of possibility, each entailing the logical one. For instance, some situations that are logically possible may be physically impossible. Since revising logical or even physical laws is no easy task, logical and physical possibilities seem to be concepts independent of contextual features and of specific individuals. A more subject-oriented concept of possibility is, instead, epistemic possibility, which in the literature has been proposed in various versions: a simple one, for example, merely

---

[1] A few exceptions are provided by Vihla (1999), who focuses on the linguistic use of modalities in medicine, by Sadegh-Zadeh (2012), who examines some logical aspects of modalities in clinical reasoning, and by Rocci (2005), who developed his views on communicative modality.

[2] When modalities of different kinds are combined in a formal system, that system is called "multimodal".

states that 'it is epistemically possible that p within a community' only if no one in that community knows that p is false; a more complex and plausible definition states that 'p is epistemically possible' means that p is not known to be false, nor would any practicable investigations establish that it is false (Hacking 1967). As appears evident from such definitions, epistemic possibility is conceived as a situated notion holding in a specific context.[3]

I note that epistemic possibility and other epistemic aspects of clinical practice play a key role in determining the main features of clinical possibility, given the association between clinical conditions and practicable interventions and investigations. The concept of clinical possibility is often involved in clinical reasoning, e.g. "reported blood in stools, with a history of weight loss, pain, and a palpated mass suggest a *possible* colorectal cancer. Rectosigmoidoscopy, biopsy and a full radiological work-up will be needed to rule out or to confirm this working diagnosis" (Sadegh-Zadeh 2012, p. 153). The concept of clinical possibility seems also to present a situated nature. A mere clinical possibility which cannot be actualised in a specific context does not seem to play an essential role in the clinical setting. In fact, only the possibilities which can be actualised seem to have, *prima facie*, the potential to provide care to patients. In this sense, clinical possibility is a teleological notion, aimed at enhancing individuals' health condition by means of specific healthcare interventions. Thus, there is a connection between clinical possibility and related healthcare interventions, which implies, from a modal point of view, a relation between clinical possibility and its potentiality of becoming actual by means of clinical interventions.[4]

Evans (2003) pointed out that healthcare interventions can be evaluated by considering the clinical notions of *effectiveness*, *appropriateness* and *feasibility*. According to him, the *effectiveness* concerns the applicability of the findings of experimental research to a target population; *appropriateness* refers to the adequacy of an intervention from the patient's perspective; and the *feasibility* of an intervention concerns conditions related to the environment in which the treatment might be implemented. I stress that these three perspectives can highlight the notion of clinical possibility, once the connection between clinical modalities and the evaluation of healthcare interventions is recognised. These possibilities, which are in fact related to effective, appropriate and feasible interventions, can be actualised, thus becoming 'real' clinical possibilities that support different therapeutic options. However, we can also identify certain situations in which the clinician makes arguments that involve the notion of 'mere' clinical possibility, whose potentiality is not guaranteed to become actual.

The main aim of this chapter is to provide some lines of reasoning for analysing the notion of clinical possibility and its connections with other related kinds of possibility.

---

[3]Interest in the notion of possibility has been recently manifested also in technology (Poser 2009). Unlike logical and physical possibility, technological possibility is about what is possible in a specific spatial and temporal context, resembling in this sense epistemic possibility (Record 2013).

[4]We do not endorse the view that all clinical possibilities are always associated with at least one treatment, since there may be possibilities which become actual as a result of no treatment.

First, the notion of clinical possibility is examined in relation to the effectiveness of treatments, to their appropriateness and their feasibility. Then, a specific section explores some basic views on the notion of possibility which may match clinical possibility, showing their validity and limitations. Finally, some concluding remarks that shed light on the normative dimension of clinical possibility are discussed.

6.2 Clinical Possibility and Effectiveness

Clinical evidence shapes the range of possibilities regarding interventions, which are relevant for clinical practice. According to the strength of evidence, a treatment may or may not be a therapeutic option. However, evidence alone does not guarantee that a new intervention can be implemented into clinical practice. It is quite standard in epidemiology to differentiate between the *efficacy* and the *effectiveness* of a clinical study (Rothman et al. 2008). The *efficacy* refers to the beneficial effect of a treatment in an experimental context, such as a randomised controlled trial (RCT). An RCT is a real experiment that modifies reality, and not just a mere description or observation of reality. Some eligibility conditions that express stringent inclusion and exclusion criteria should be followed in order to recruit a sample of patients in the arms of the clinical trial. Other clinical features should also be fulfilled that go according to the design and aims of the trial. Given these strict experimental and controlled conditions, it is assumed that well designed RCTs tend to be internally valid. Internal validity is a measure of how much the differences between groups are due to a specific treatment rather than to other factors. And yet, RCTs tend to provide somewhat amplified results compared to those obtained in daily practice. Such tendency for amplification is a threat for external validity (Carthwright 2007), that is to say, evidence applied outside the experimental context may not result in the same level of *effectiveness*. Hence, the effectiveness of an intervention indicates whether it works in clearly defined conditions, expressing the level of benefits *versus* harm and clarifying who will benefit from its use (Evans 2003).

When considering effectiveness, many constraints such as biological possibility as well as epistemic and non-epistemic limitations seem to have an impact on clinical possibility. The epistemic dimension related to the design of epidemiological studies can, in fact, corroborate or exclude new clinical possibilities. Moreover, clinical possibility should also be based on biological possibility, related to knowledge of the pathophysiological mechanisms involved in the clinical discourse. Whatever opposes accepted biological knowledge is ruled out as a clinical possibility. In addition, non-epistemic limitations associated, for instance, with the ethical and legal requirements of clinical research further shape the notion of clinical possibility (Emanuel et al. 2000). Clinical possibilities may be further restricted by ethical principles and criteria orientating clinical practice.

Clinical evidence obtained from experimental studies may be reduced or unconfirmed in a context of practical applicability. A similar argument holds for the notion of clinical possibility. Worrall (2002) pointed out that randomisation in a trial does not exclude the possibility of incurring biases, confounding factors and paradoxes. On the other hand, studies called "pragmatic", i.e. not randomised and more easily applicable in clinical practice, play a key role in confirming or refuting the effectiveness of a treatment (Bluhm 2009). Thus, evidence belonging to pragmatic studies may significantly contribute towards deciding on the best interventions to be applied to a specific population.

6.3   Clinical Possibility and Appropriateness

Beyond the internal and external validity of a clinical intervention, evidence for clinical practice needs to be clinically appropriate. Appropriateness evaluates interventions from the patient's perspective. In fact, interventions are defined as appropriate when they are consistent with individualized aspects of care, based on the patient's experiences, expectations and values (Shapiro 2010). Many patients receive inappropriate or unnecessary care, leading to an overuse or underuse of healthcare practices (Hicks 1994). There is therefore a need to propose methodological tools so as to determine the proper level of appropriateness for patients. Not all treatments which are both internally and externally valid are deemed appropriate when applied to a single clinical case. Likewise, some clinical possibilities holding at population level may not apply to a specific context. It seems however reasonable to assume that, in pragmatic studies, evidence is more likely to be shaped by different individual decisions rather than by experimental research.

I have pointed out that the notion of clinical possibility is involved in the diagnostic process. For instance, when making a differential diagnosis, it is important to take into account a finite and precise set of clinical possibilities so as to rule out those that express incorrect diagnostic hypotheses. At this stage, differential diagnosis may be used to isolate a specific clinical hypothesis, even if it was not present in the set of initial possibilities and there is no certainty as to whether it is the correct one. Alternatively, if evidence exists to positively confirm one of the initial hypotheses, then differential diagnosis may ascertain the presence of a specific disease, ruling out other possibilities (Federspil 2004).

Clinical possibilities may be positively supported by both a *scintilla of evidence* or the conflict with the epistemic and non-epistemic limitations mentioned above. Although possibilities which are positively confirmed by evidence are essential in the clinical context, in some limited cases even those possibilities not receiving direct and positive confirmation prove to be relevant to clinical practice. In fact, there may be complex situations in which bodily signs, morphological and laboratory examinations do not suffice to make a diagnosis. In such situations, the clinician may use the criterion of *ex juvantibus*, e.g. to choose a drug with a demonstrated effectiveness for a specific disease. If mitigation of signs appears or there is even healing, then the original diagnostic hypothesis may be confirmed. In other words, the *ex juvantibus* diagnostic criterion states that the observed beneficial effectiveness of a treatment—if a diagnostic hypothesis has been formulated—may lead to a partial confirmation of the original hypothesis. Instead, if there was no diagnostic hypothesis at all, then the set of signs and symptoms would have to be resolved without any diagnosis. Thus, even those possibilities which are not directly supported by evidence may play a role in clinical practice, if they are actualised by some diagnostic method. In most cases, however, such a possibility of becoming actual (potentiality) is a distinctive feature of clinical possibility. I argue that potentiality is in fact connected with the teleological dimension of clinical knowledge.[5] In situations in which there is no treatment of demonstrated utility for the patient afflicted with an incurable disease, a mere possibility, even when not confirmed by a *scintilla of evidence*, can be taken into account by the clinician, as long as it is consistent with biological, ethical, legal and technological constraints.

6.4   Clinical Possibility and Feasibility

The feasibility of interventions is a key issue for clinical possibility. All possibilities that are associated with hypotheses supporting feasible clinical interventions can be actualised and become 'real' clinical possibilities. The concept of feasibility is inherently normative because it refers to interventions which *can* and *should* be implemented for the treatment of patients' diseases. Feasibility concerns the evaluation of the viability of a clinical intervention for which there is insufficient consensus on the proposed intervention's clinical value in a specific context. In the literature, feasibility has been associated with the following questions regarding the implementation of a new intervention: "Can it work? Does it work? Will it work?" (Bowen et al 2009). The first question can be addressed by experimental or pragmatic studies, whose validity and limitations have been already pointed out. The second question may refer to studies called "proof of concept", which examine the possibility of testing the intervention in a full-scale trial later on. This is the case, for example, with Phase I or Phase II studies in pharmacology (pilot studies). After assessing the possible harmfulness of a drug, its proper dosage for humans and its initial desirable clinical activity, full-scale Phase III trials can be carried out. Early-phase studies are also used to make decisions on some statistical features of Phase III trials, such as power, effect size and sample size. Finally, let us move on to the third question ("will it work?"), which takes on the most important notion of feasibility. This last sense focusses in fact on the conditions in which clinical interventions can and should be implemented in a specific environment (Evans 2003). A treatment is feasible, in this sense, if it can be implemented with the resources available within a determined context. The key constraints associated with the feasibility of an intervention are mainly due to economic issues. Various forms of economic evaluation of healthcare interventions (e.g. cost benefits, cost effectiveness, cost consequences, cost utility,

---

[5]This issue will be later explained when presenting some basic views on the notion of clinical possibility.

etc.) lead to decisions regarding the possibility of starting an intervention in a particular context (Drummond et al 2005). However, also social and cultural attitudes may play a non-secondary role concerning the feasibility of interventions.

The importance of potentiality conditions expresses the purpose-fulfilment nature of clinical possibility, which in fact, has to do with choosing interventions and achieving certain clinical goals. Potentiality should not be wholly identified with mere possibility: something is potential if there exist some essential conditions that may make it become actual. However, as potentiality implies mere possibility and not vice versa, these two notions must not be confused. If something is actual, then it is already possible. A potential condition must be compatible with a specific context in order to become actual, whereas there is no guarantee that mere possibilities may become actual. We have argued that clinical possibilities are, with few exceptions, potentialities, and this fact is associated with the importance of the feasibility of interventions in clinical practice. That is, those possibilities which may be actualised by means of a treatment play a major role in clinical practice.

The notion of 'health potential' has recently been proposed in the literature to stress the usefulness of the concept of potentiality in the clinical context (Chiffi and Zanotti 2015; Zanotti and Chiffi 2015). As we have seen, health potential is associated with the possibility of enhancing the health status of patients, in view of their actual clinical condition, by means of effective, appropriate and feasible interventions. This concept seems to be particularly suitable for nursing practice, since the need to assess the maximum level of achievable *self-care* for a single patient is one of the main goals of nursing. Determining the potentiality of *self-care* is the basis for nursing interventions and may make a critical difference between the medical and nursing fields. Medical interventions are required when there is an alteration from a given physiological norm, whereas nursing interventions are required when a patient's self-care is not at an optimal level of potential.

6.5   Some Basic Views on the Nature of Clinical Possibility

In this section, I present three fundamental perspectives on the semantic and ontological nature of possibility which may turn out to be relevant to our discourse on the nature of clinical possibility. These perspectives are: (a) *possible world semantics*, (b) *possibility theory* and (c) the *theory of dispositional possibility*. Although such views may be associated with other and more specific modal theories, they can still provide deep insights into some basic properties of possibility.

A classical and well-known approach to modalities is that of *possible world semantics* (originated by Kripke 1959). It is commonly assumed that things may be different in many ways. Intuitively, a possible world is an exhaustive and coherent scenario, which might represent a different way in which the actual world exists. Alternatively, a possible world might also be completely different from our actual world. In standard possible world semantics used in modal logic, proposition p is possible only if there exists at least a possible world achievable by a specific accessibility relation (expressing a property of mathematical relations such as reflexivity, transitivity, etc.) for which the proposition holds true. Proposition p is necessary only if p is true in all accessible possible worlds. Possible world semantics has been used to handle possibility from a qualitative perspective. Many metaphysical doctrines have been associated with a possible world view on modalities such as *modal realism* (all possible worlds are as real as the one we live in even if such worlds are not in a causal relation with the actual world) (Lewis 1973), *ersatzism*[6] (only one world really exists, i.e. the actual one; possible worlds are merely surrogate notions) (Stalnaker 2003), and so forth. Therefore, even if there is no close connection between possible world semantics and a specific metaphysical claim on the nature of modalities, according to a possible world view there may exist (or be postulated at least) coherent and complete scenarios expressing ways in which things might be.

Beyond the possible world perspective on modal notions, I consider a second view of the nature of possibility. When dealing with a situated notion, it may be more correct to speak of "degrees of possibilities" in relation to concepts such as health, disease or healing, which some authors consider to be vague. For instance, the attribution of a degree of probability to the vague notion of health may face methodological limitations, since the concept itself seems to present undefined borders. A possible alternative in which to handle such indefinite notions consists in attributing to them some degrees of possibility. This idea corresponds with the mathematical structure of "possibility theory", inspired by the systems of fuzzy sets and logic (Zadeh 1999). A fuzzy set is a collection of objects with grades of membership, i.e. there are no sharp boundaries between members and non-members of the collection.[7] A possibility distribution represents the state of knowledge of an agent assessing what is plausible from what is less plausible, and distinguishing the normal course of events from what is not. This distribution is a function from state of things S to an ordered scale L with a top value 1 (expressing full possibility) and a bottom value 0 (impossibility). I shall not examine here the formal apparatus of possibility theory, since what is of importance for our discourse is the fact that a *situated* and *quantitative* notion of possibility is used in clinical practice when dealing with vague clinical notions.[8] When the idea of degrees of possibility is involved, a mathematical structure that is different from possible world semantics can be built, enabling us to model vague clinical notions that involve clinical possibilities. Indeed, clinical possibility is directed towards the care of a specific individual and is related to a definite context. Thus, according to this second view of modalities, also a quantitative notion of possibility seems to be involved in clinical practice, and not just a qualitative one. Conversely, if we focus on clinical impossibilities, we may note that some of

---

[6]From the German word "*Ersatz*", meaning "substitute" or "surrogate".

[7]For a detailed analysis clarifying the application of possibility theory and fuzzy sets to medicine, see (Sadegh-Zadeh 2000, 2012).

[8]It should be recognized that qualitative forms of possibility may also be represented by possibility theory. Moreover, it is worth noting that the connection between agent's states of knowledge and possibility theory supports an epistemic view on possibility.

them remain absolute, since they violate logical or physical/biological constraints. In fact, other clinical impossibilities are merely contingent and may be converted into new viable possibilities as soon as innovative clinical discoveries or technological innovations create new possibilities. However, one may argue that the difficulties of dealing with the concepts of health and disease do not only depend on the fuzziness of these notions, but also on their normative status. Therefore, the possibility associated with the notion of health and disease may be considered as a deontic modality, i.e. a qualitative notion of possibility related to what *should* be done in order to restore, maintain or enhance the *normal* status of a person's health. Following this view, the quantitative perspective on clinical possibility is not suitable.

Now let us look into the third view on the nature of clinical possibility. The above-mentioned notion of health potential seems to share some ideas with the recently developed theory of *dispositional possibility* (Borghini and Williams 2008). Dispositions are properties assigned to entities which manifest themselves only in specific conditions. In this context, possibility refers to the existence of a specific disposition that might manifest itself, given some stimulus conditions. For instance, a glass expresses the disposition to shatter when struck. In applying dispositions to clinical practice, we focus on those known dispositions that show a causal power. Mumford (2003) has pointed out that dispositions are poor causal explanations that not always clearly express the underlying mechanisms involved in the explanation.

Unlike a possible world view on the notion of possibility, a dispositional perspective on modalities suitable for clinical practice holds that there is only one world (the actual one), which counts with many dispositions that may become actual. Other worlds are not even postulated. Again, unlike a perspective of clinical possibility based on the degrees of possibility, the dispositional view considers possibility as a qualitative notion. In a dispositional view of modalities, in fact, there is no interest in possibilities not involving any kind of relation with the actual world (significantly called 'alien possibilities'). Only those possibilities which express a tendency in the actual world towards a given (health/disease) condition are considered, ruling out the alien ones. Such range restriction may be advantageous when addressing the issue of possibility within the clinical setting.

Dispositions in the health context have a functional dimension and contribute to achieving a fitness value of the organism, given certain conditions. The disposition of the heart to pump blood, for example, is associated with the possibility of keeping the blood circulating due to cardiac contractions activated by a flow of electricity. If this electrical flow is altered, the heart's reduced capacity to pump correctly causes disturbances in its rhythm, eventually resulting in blood circulation. The dispositional view of clinical possibility also seems to have some problems. The nature of clinical possibility cannot be wholly specified by the main features of functional dispositions. It is not possible, in fact, to identify the set of clinical possibilities with function-oriented possibilities related to pathophysiological knowledge, since ethical, social, and technological constrains can also shape clinical possibility.

6.6 Conclusions

An analysis of the foundational aspects of clinical possibility may represent a new line of research in the philosophy of health care. Although modal concepts are widely used in clinical reasoning, a philosophical debate on such notions is still at an initial stage. I did not present here a specific thesis regarding the problem of defining clinical possibility: I have suggested that clinical reasoning should contemplate possibilities even when not merely related to functional pathophysiological aspects; moreover, I have provided some elements of analysis of clinical possibility as a distinctive kind of modality. I have then outlined the limitations arising when one considers the basic views on the nature of clinical possibility.

I described how clinical possibility is shaped by different kinds of possibilities, reason why such a notion is particularly difficult to analyse. In some cases, mere clinical possibilities can be used in clinical practice, e.g. the *ex juvantibus* criterion. I have also clarified that the possibilities which express the potential of enhancing a health state seem to count as 'real' clinical possibilities. A distinction has been proposed between possibilities supported by at least a *scintilla of evidence* and others for which there is no positive evidence in their support. It has been stated that a mere possibility, even if not confirmed by a *scintilla of evidence*, may play a key role in clinical reasoning when other options of care are absent. Even these kinds of possibilities should not be held as *alien possibilities*, i.e. totally unrelated to the actual world: in fact, further clinical research might provide evidence confirming a mere possibility related to the actual world. However, it is not always possible to know in advance whether a possibility, without any confirming evidence at the time, is alien or not. I then examined how analysis of the *effectiveness*, *appropriateness* and *feasibility* of clinical treatments may highlight some specific features of clinical possibility which would be difficult to deal with otherwise. I specify the role of possibilities which may be actualised within the clinical context in order to enhance patients' health condition and develop what I call their "health potential".

Subsequently, I examine three basic perspectives of the semantics and nature of possibility, *possible world semantics, possibility theory* and the *theory of dispositional possibility*. These perspectives assume that the notion of possibility may be qualitative or quantitative, absolute or situated, normative or descriptive. I argue that none of these perspectives seems to express the main features of clinical possibility, which all the more suggests that a foundational analysis of such notion is still a *desideratum*. I am convinced that clinical possibility cannot merely be equated with biological or pathophysiological possibilities, since both epistemic (objectivity of clinical knowledge, error reduction, etc.) and non-epistemic values (ethical, legal issues, etc.) in clinical practice may shape the range of possibility in this context.[9]

It seems plausible to assume that clinical possibility itself is a normative notion rather than an alethic one because of the normative dimension of values in shaping

---

[9]For a clear-cut analysis regarding the role of epistemic and non-epistemic values in scientific enterprise, see (Risjord 2014). For the possibility of defining some kinds of modality in terms of other modalities, see (Fine 2002).

clinical possibility. This view may be clearer if we focus on the notion of necessity, defined in logic as "not possible not". It is usually accepted that alethic necessity is *factive* (i.e. the logical operator for necessity as well as, for instance, the knowledge operator lead to the truth of the necessitated (or known) proposition); whereas the concept of "being obligatory" according to a norm is not factive, since norms can be violated. If there is a norm stating that it is obligatory to pay taxes, it does not follow that everyone pays taxes. Similar to normative modalities, clinical necessity seems not to be factive,[10] which would point to clinical possibility being (at least *prima facie*) a normative modality. A situation can be clinically possible not because it is merely directed towards the notion of truth, but because it must fulfil norms of biological and pathophysiological plausibility as well as moral and legal correctness or evidential support. I uphold the claim that these values contribute towards the constitution of clinical possibility.

Further lines of research may provide conceptual frameworks linking clinical modalities, therapeutic reasoning and clinical practice.

References

Bluhm, R.: Some observations on "observational" research. Perspect. Biol. Med. **52**(2), 252–263 (2009)

Borghini, A., Williams, N.E.: A dispositional theory of possibility. Dialectica **62**(1), 21–41 (2008)

Bowen, D.J., Kreuter, M., Spring, B., et al.: How we design feasibility studies. Am. J. Prev. Med. **36**(5), 452–457 (2009)

Cartwright, N.: Are RCTs the gold standard? Biosocieties **2**(1), 11–20 (2007)

Chiffi, D., Zanotti, R.: Medical and nursing diagnoses: a critical comparison. J. Eval. Clin. Pract. **21**(1), 1–6 (2015)

Drummond, M.F., Sculpher, M.J., Torrance, W.G., O'Brien, B.J., Stoddart, G.L.: Methods for the Economic Evaluation of Health Care Programmes. Oxford University Press, Oxford (2005)

Emanuel, E.J., Wendler, D., Grady, C.: What makes clinical research ethical? J. Am. Med. Assoc. **283**(20), 2701–2711 (2000)

Evans, D.: Hierarchy of evidence: a framework for ranking evidence evaluating healthcare interventions. J. Clin. Nurs. **12**(1), 77–84 (2003)

Federspil, G.: Logica clinica: i principi del metodo in medicina. McGraw-Hill, Milan (2004)

Feinstein, A.R.: Clin. Biostat. Mosby, St. Louis (1977)

Fine, K.: The varieties of necessity. In: Gendler, T.S., Hawthorne, J. (eds.) Conceivability and Possibility, pp. 253–282. Oxford University Press, Oxford (2002)

Hacking, I.: Possibility. Philos. Rev. **76**(2), 143–168 (1967)

Hicks, N.R.: Some observations on attempts to measure appropriateness of care. BMJ **309**(6956), 730–733 (1994)

Kripke, S.A.: A completeness theorem in modal logic. J. Symbol. Log. **24**(01), 1–14 (1959)

Lewis, D.: Counterfactuals. Basil Blackwell, Oxford (1973)

Mumford, S.: Dispositions. Oxford University Press, Oxford (2003)

---

[10] Notice that the failure of *factivity* (corresponding to the failure of the reflexive accessibility relation in a possible world semantics) for clinical necessity may provide only an indication of its similarities with normative modalities. This is not a complete and independent argument for the normativity of clinical modalities, but just a conjecture.

Poser, H.: Technology and necessity. Monist **92**(3), 441–451 (2009)

Proudfoot, M., Lacey, A.R.: Routledge Dictionary of Philosophy, 4th edn. Routledge, New York (2009)

Record, I.: Technology and epistemic possibility. J. Gen. Philos. Sci. **44**(2), 319–336 (2013)

Risjord, M.: Philosophy of Social Science: A Contemporary Introduction. Routledge, New York (2014)

Rocci, A.: La modalità epistemica tra semantica e argomentazione. ISU Università Cattolica, Milan (2005)

Rothman, K.J., Greenland, S., Lash, T.L. (eds.): Modern Epidemiology. Lippincott Williams & Wilkins, Philadelphia (2008)

Sadegh-Zadeh, K.: Fuzzy health, illness, and disease. J. Med. Philos. **25**(5), 605–638 (2000)

Sadegh-Zadeh, K.: Handbook of Analytic Philosophy of Medicine, vol. 113. Springer, Dordrecht (2012)

Shapiro, S.E.: Grading evidence for practice. Adv. Emerg. Nurs. J. **32**(1), 59–67 (2010)

Stalnaker, R.: Ways a World Might Be: Metaphysical and Anti-Metaphysical Essays. Oxford University Press, Oxford (2003)

Vihla, M.: Medical Writing: Modality in Focus. Rodopi, Amsterdam (1999)

Worrall, J.: What evidence in evidence-based medicine?. Philos. Sci. **69**(S3):S316–S330 (2002)

Zadeh, L.A.: Fuzzy sets as a basis for a theory of possibility. Fuzzy Sets Syst. **100**, 9–34 (1999)

Zanotti, R., Chiffi, D.: Diagnostic frameworks and nursing diagnoses: a normative stance. Nurs. Philos. **16**(1), 64–73 (2015)

Chapter 7
The Epistemology of Placebo Effect

7.1 Introduction

The present chapter focuses on the interplay between the epistemological dimension of beliefs associated with the notions of "placebo" and "placebo effect" and their therapeutic value. Unfortunately, these medical concepts of placebo and placebo effect lack an adequate level of conceptual clarity (Miller and Brody 2011). Many attempts have been made to explicate these concepts, but there is no general agreement in medicine or in philosophy about their definitions (see for example Grünbaum 1984; Brody 2000; Giaretta 2013). As stated by Brody (2000), defining these concepts in a logically consistent way is difficult, perhaps impossible, since terms usually associated with placebo such as "inert" or "non-specific" seem to be misleading. There may be in fact placebos that are active while their effect may be specific (Howick 2011). Our aim is not to provide a new explication for the concept of "placebo" or "placebo effect", but rather to analyse their intuitive use in the construction of important examples for the analysis of knowledge (Nozick 1981; Kripke 2011). On the one hand, quite unexpectedly, an epistemological analysis of beliefs associated with placebo may reveal key features for the notions of placebo and placebo effect as used in clinical research and practice. On the other hand, the clinical use of these concepts may suggest new critical reflection of the nature of knowledge associated with placebo-based beliefs. This type of belief is usually supposed to be self-fulfilling: the patient is cured simply because he believes to be cured (Johansson and Lynøe 2008). As we shall see in the next sections, it is commonly assumed, especially in epistemology, that the truth of a placebo-based belief would merely require the patient to hold such a belief. I will point out that this perspective may be misleading in a multi-agent context, where placebo-based beliefs are justified by higher-order beliefs that are essentially influenced by the clinical context in which (even "dummy") treatments are administered. Placebo-based beliefs are, in fact, contextual, since they are

D. Chiffi, *Clinical Reasoning: Knowledge, Uncertainty, and Values in Health Care*,
Studies in Applied Philosophy, Epistemology and Rational Ethics 58,
https://doi.org/10.1007/978-3-030-59094-9_7

instantiated in a specific clinical setting composed of the environment, doctor-patient beliefs, interaction and communication.[1] Their nature is not merely internal because they also require interaction with the external world; and the justification of beliefs according to internal or external methods is a key issue in epistemology. This is precisely why epistemologists have focused their attention on placebo-based beliefs.

Section 7.2 is devoted to an analysis and a short review of the main methodological issues related to placebo trials in clinical research. Section 7.3 explores the epistemological nature of placebo-based beliefs in light of the analysis of propositional knowledge made by Nozick (1981) and Kripke (2011). In Sect. 7.4, the alleged self-fulfilling nature of placebo-based beliefs is analysed. Section 7.5 makes some concluding remarks.

7.2   Placebo and Treatments in Clinical Research

In clinical research, placebos are used in the control group of a trial in order to evaluate the therapeutic effect of a new drug or therapy. However, if an already available effective treatment exists, "the doctor will wish to know whether a new treatment is more, or less, effective than the old, not that it is more effective than nothing" (Hill 1963, p. 1048; Worrall 2010). In the light of Hill's remark, Rothman (1996) highlights the problem regarding comparisons between treatments and placebos in clinical research.

> Suppose you had an old friend Bill, who you knew was tall, and a new friend Bob, who also seems tall. You wish to find out how tall Bob is in relation to Bill. Most people would ask Bill and Bob to stand back to back and measure the vertical difference between the tops of their heads. Suppose that Bill and Bob are not in the same place. You can use a tape to measure Bill's height first, then visit Bob and measure his height, and then compare the two heights. (Rothman 1996, pp. 3–4)

The direct and indirect methods of measuring are equivalent only in ideal conditions. If, for instance, Bob and Bill are not in the same place and we do not have a precise device for measuring at our disposal, then the direct and indirect methods are not practically equivalent. You can state that either Bill or Bob is tall, but you cannot know with precision who is taller. Placebo controlled trials (PCTs) are designed to evaluate whether a treatment is better than a placebo, but it may furnish very little information as to what extent that treatment is effective and better than other already known treatments. The purpose of PCTs is not to understand why a placebo works, but to show whether a certain treatment works better than the placebo (Benedetti 2009). Yet, there are some properly designed studies that make an analysis of how the placebo group compares with both the treatment and no-treatment groups, and show the therapeutic effect of various forms of the placebo (e.g. the effect of different colours of placebo-pills on a patient's health and beliefs) (de Craen et al. 1996).

---

[1] Empirical research must determine the aspects of the clinical context that are relevant to therapy.

Rothman (1996) states that, when the comparison is made with a group of patients receiving placebo in a PCT, the study does not need to be very large in order to assess statistically significant findings.[2] Unfortunately, if this is so, then our measure of the effect may show large confidence intervals. In the aforementioned example, it would be similar to a visual assessment of the heights of Bill and Bob, which can only lead to state that one is shorter or taller than the other, without providing any further specifications of their heights. It is worth noting however that the use of placebo does not provide a baseline measure to evaluate the effect of a treatment, since placebo responses express a high degree of variability among individuals (Benedetti 2009). This would equate to measuring Bill's and Bob's heights starting from different reference points. In addition, there are no specific regulations on the constituents of the placebos and, consequently, placebos may vary considerably across trials (Golom 1995). But problems may also arise when the direct method is applied, as happens in 'active' controlled trials (ACTs), in which a new treatment is compared with one with a demonstrated beneficial effect for a disease. ACTs are of course necessarily applied when there are ethical limitations to using placebos in place of an already known effective treatment. From a methodological viewpoint, there may be different types of standard supporting care for a specific disease and, in some cases, it may be difficult to find a 'gold standard' comparator (Tramèr et al. 1998). Moreover, there is no assurance that an ACT is effective in new experimental conditions, i.e. there is a hidden historical control assumption (Clark and Leaverton 1994). To this must be added that interpreting the findings of no difference between a new treatment and the ACT as evidence of the efficacy for the new treatment, may be misleading if we do not take into account the confidence intervals of the effect of both treatments without considering that of the effect of a placebo arm. The three confidence intervals may in fact overlap (Makuch and Johnson 1989). In this case, without a placebo arm, there may be no clear grounds for stating that a new treatment is effective. At any rate, it is necessary not to reduce the placebo effect to the result of a placebo arm in a trial, since many other features may shape findings of this arm, e.g. regression towards the mean, natural history of a disease, etc. Indeed, it seems that both PCTs and ACTs have some *pros* and *cons*, and deciding on which one to use may depend on the nature of the specific treatment to be tested.

All in all, the concepts of placebo and placebo effect are difficult to define and the fruitfulness of the applications of these concepts in an intuitive sense raises many methodological questions. This may be a clue of the lack of an adequate epistemological study on these notions and on the nature of beliefs associated with them.

---

[2]For a different view, see Howick (2009).

7.3 Beliefs on Placebo and the Analysis of Knowledge

In the previous section, the concept of placebo has been analysed by indicating some epistemological considerations raised by its use in clinical research. Quite surprisingly, the concept of placebo has been used in order to clarify the philosophical notion of propositional knowledge, specifically to provide a counterexample to Nozick's (1981) analysis of propositional knowledge, also called the "tracking theory of knowledge". Nozick lists four conditions which he claims are jointly necessary and sufficient to analyse propositional knowledge. He tries to connect truth and belief, so as to avoid Gettier (1963) type objections to knowledge as "justified true beliefs".[3] Nozick's Analysis of Knowledge (NAK) is the following:

A subject S knows the proposition p if and only if.

(1) p is true
(2) S believes that p
(3) If p weren't true, S wouldn't believe that p
(4) If p were true, S would believe that p.[4]

When the above conditions hold, we may *track* the fact that p. Conditions 3 and 4 make use of subjective conditionals; that is, conditionals using verbs in a subjective, and not in an indicative mood, e.g. "If p were true, q would be true". This conditional is evaluated as true when q is true in the *p-neighbourhood* of the actual world. The *p-neighbourhood* is the set of those possible worlds that are considered close to the actual world. However, Nozick (1981) does not fully explicate the concept of closeness among worlds.[5] It has been pointed out that NAK presents some nice properties capable of stopping many sceptical arguments (Luper-Foy 1984), even though the epistemic closure principle does not hold, since knowing that p is true does not convey us the knowledge of its logical consequences, that is to say, in logical terms knowledge is closed under known entailment (Yamada 2014).

Because of the possible redundancy that can be derived from the above conditions[6] and some counterexamples to NAK, Nozick slightly modified his conditions for analysing knowledge (see later). Some counterexamples to NAK come from "self-fulfilling beliefs": a belief that p is self-fulfilling when it turns out to be true *just*

---

[3] A classical text on the notions of knowledge and belief is (Hintikka 1962). An influencing collection of papers on the theory of knowledge is (Moser 2005).

[4] Of course, in the case of logical or mathematical truths which are usually considered necessary, their knowledge may rule out condition (3) as redundant.

[5] Nozick describes the semantics of subjective conditionals in the following way: For any possible worlds w_1 and w_2, w_2 is in the p neighborhood of w_1 if and only if p is true in w_2 and there are no worlds wp and $w\neg p$ such that: (1) p is true in wp and false in $w\neg p$; (2) $w\neg p$ is closer to w_1 than w_2 is to w_1; (3) wp is at least as close to w_1 as $w\neg p$ is to w_1. $A \rightarrow B$ is true at w if and only if B is true in the A neighborhood of w. (see Nozick 1981, 680–681, n8). Intuitively, the p-neighborhood of w is the largest path of worlds where p is true; and it is uninterrupted by any world where p is false that is closest to w (Comesaña 2007).

[6] Notice that independently of the accepted theory of counterfactual, it is usually assumed that counterfactual implication entails classical implication. If this is assumed, Kripke (2011) has shown that some redundancies are derivable by NAK.

because an individual believes it. Let us imagine a patient who believes she will recover and therefore does recover. Suppose that condition 3 is fulfilled, i.e. if it were true, the patient would believe it (there is no other way of regaining health except by holding such a belief). In this case, it is unclear whether condition 3 holds or not; that is, if the proposition stating that if the patient will recover were not true, would the patient not believe it? Nozick (1981) states that this seems to be a case of truth tracking a belief, not of a belief tracking the truth. In this example, according to Nozick, it seems more likely that believing p implies p, rather than its converse. In the case of self-fulfilling beliefs, Nozick (1981, p. 196) leaves open the possibility that (i) both 3 and 4 do not hold; (ii) we add to NAK the condition "not-(not believing $p \rightarrow$ not-p)"; or (iii) it is not the case that 3 or 4 hold solely: at least one condition between 3 or 4 must hold. Condition 4 seems not to be particularly problematic, because if I can recover *only* by holding a placebo-based belief, then my recovering is completely due to my believing it. In Nozick's example, in fact, there is no other *method* of recovering except by holding such a belief. Instead, what may be problematic in the case of self-fulfilling beliefs is condition 3, since from not-p does not seem always intuitively valid to conclude to not-believing p. For instance, if p means "I will recover", from the fact that I will not recover does not seem to follow *in any case* my disbelief that I will recover. The method related to placebo effect does not seem to play any role here. Therefore, the options (i)–(iii) suggested by Nozick are not fully relevant for analysing self-fulfilling beliefs. What is (at least partially) missing in Nozick's picture at this stage is an analysis of the methods capable of providing epistemic grounds for beliefs. More generally, Nozick proposes the following argument for placebo beliefs (NAPB), which he assumes to be a special case of self-fulfilling beliefs:

(NAPB 1) truth is usually different from what we believe about it, whereas believing that a placebo effect is efficacious helps to make it so. Given this fact, there might be a different account of truth (and therefore of knowledge) for those truths which are belief-dependent or, alternatively (Nozick 2001, p. 47).

(NAPB 2) we might base our concept of truth as simply independent of our beliefs (Nozick 2001, p. 318, n 64).

Thus, it seems that beliefs such as those associated with the placebo effect impose a severe epistemological reflection on the interplay between truth and belief, since they are not in complete accordance with NAK. But it is also important to note that beliefs that are not considered self-fulfilling may also provide counterexamples to NAK. Let us examine this further example: "A grandmother sees her grandson is well when he comes to visit; but if he were sick or dead, others would tell her he was well to spare her upset" (Nozick 1981, p. 179). In this case, even though the grandmother violates condition 3, she comes to know that her grandson is well. In the light of these kinds of problems, Nozick proposed a new fine-grained analysis of knowledge referring to a specific method (M) as follows:

Nozick's Revisited Analysis of Knowledge (NRAK).

(1°) p is true
(2°) S believes, via method M, that p.
(3°) If p weren't true and S were to use M to arrive at a belief whether (or not) p, then S wouldn't believe, via M, that p. (*Sensitivity condition*)
(4°) If p were true and S were to use M to arrive at a belief whether (or not) then S would believe, via M, that p (*Adherence condition*) (Nozick 1981, p. 179).

Nozick invites us to consider yet another example based on the notion of placebo in order to evaluate NRAK. Let us observe first that there are scientific results showing that it is possible to obtain a placebo effect in clinical research and practice even without deception, i.e. even when the patient knows that the substance administered is a placebo.[7] For instance, open-label placebo has been evaluated superior to a no-treatment group in a randomized controlled trial in irritable bowel syndrome (Kaptchuk et al. 2010). Nozick (1981, p. 561) imagines a situation in which a patient is aware of the scientific findings associated with administering an open-label placebo and in fact receives a placebo of this kind. According to Nozick, the knowledge of the effect of the placebo would be "ungrounded", since the psychophysiological mechanisms of *this* placebo would be activated *merely* by this *specific* self-fulfilling belief: this would be the case of a reflexive belief. If one asks: "Why do you hold this belief"? One answer based on reflexive beliefs would be as we have already seen: "Because I believe this belief", which would seem to be an implausible answer even if we know the therapeutic value of an open-label placebo. Nozick does not go further in investigating the case, but asks the reader to imagine the impact of this example on NRAK in order to make any refinements to his definition of knowledge. In this example, one might wonder whether the patient receiving an open-label placebo *knows* that it will have a beneficial effect due precisely to the placebo. Let p be "the patient will feel better". If p is not the case and the belief of p is precisely the method justifying this belief, then the patient would not believe p. However, in this case the belief of p is the method for supporting the belief of p itself. The belief of p turns out to be ungrounded and, therefore, it does not appear to constitute proper knowledge. It is usually viewed as a mark of irrationality to let one's beliefs be affected by what one wants to happen, or to consider the effects as evidence for them. The Kripkean analysis hereafter is devoted to exploring the possibility of employing irrational methods in NRAK.

Kripke (2011) proposed some counterexamples to NRAK, from which I consider only one. Such example makes reference to a placebo in a trial in which a "sloppy" scientist neglected to include experimental controls in the study design. Once again, Nozick's account of knowledge is evaluated by examining the relation between beliefs and placebo, although self-fulfilling beliefs are not directly involved in the Kripkean example.

---

[7] However, deception in the use of placebo is more likely to occur in clinical practice rather than in clinical research, in which the possible use of a placebo is reported in the informed consent procedure.

Consider a medical experimenter, testing the efficacy of a new drug on a certain disease. [...] Suppose he neglects to give a placebo to a control group. If his patients in fact tend to have significantly above-average recovery rates, and he concludes that he has tested a drug that is (chemically) effective against the disease, the scientific community would judge that his research is worthless (or, at least, highly inconclusive). He has not ruled out the possibility that his favorable results are due to a placebo effect. [...] Suppose, however, that in fact placebos are completely (or nearly completely) ineffective against this particular disease, although neither the experimenter nor anyone else in the medical community has any reason to suppose that this is so. (Kripke 2011, pp. 170–171)

In this example, if "p = this drug will cure this disease", we have a situation in which, if p were not true by means of M, the scientist would not believe that p. This happens because if the scientist had experimented an ineffective drug, there would have been no substantial clinical improvement for patients, as the placebo effect cannot occur for such disease. Instead, if p were true by means of M, the "sloppy" scientist would believe, via M, that p. Thus, even though Nozick's conditions 3° and 4° are satisfied, the example does not seem to express knowledge. Kripke's counterexample to NRAK is based on the assumption that only external methods can guarantee knowledge, with which I concur. Moreover, it shows that the irrationality of the methods used does not prevent satisfying all NRAK conditions.[8] A scientist's beliefs are in fact irrational and unjustified, since they do not take into consideration the correct methods used by the scientific community.

When examining Kripke's example of the "sloppy" scientist, Adams and Clarke (2005) point out that there may be two types of sloppiness: one is related to error in screening patients, i.e. false positive and false negative results in a diagnostic test, or in the experimental conditions for administering a treatment. In statistics, the errors that are important for medical diagnostics are called respectively "type I error" and "type II error".[9] However, the existence of a residual risk of error called "inductive risk" for empirical knowledge is unavoidable, since both types of errors cannot be completely eliminated (Hempel 1965). According to Adams and Clarke (2005), this is not the type of sloppiness seen in Kripke's example. The scientist's sloppiness would be associated with a lack of proper control in confirming information, and not with an error of information in itself. The authors state that Kripke's example resembles the situation in which, prior to cross-examination, a witness may be telling the truth and be perfectly reliable. One may wonder how is it possible to judge the witness as reliable before executing proper controls and cross-examinations. Adam and Clarke (2005, p. 218) write: "This does not mean that the witness was not reliable until after the cross-examination". One may reply that we do not know whether the witness would be reliable or not until after examination. The witness may be in fact reliable, but there is no way of ascertaining this properly and objectively before

---

[8]It is worth noting that Kripke's example is very abstract. In real-world situations, many other conditions in addition to the placebo effect, such as confounding factors, epidemiological paradoxes, etc., may contribute to influencing the findings of a clinical study. Of course, these real-world aspects of epidemiological research do not weaken the epistemological value and beauty of Kripke's counterexample to NRAK.

[9]A connection between type I and type II statistical errors and conditions 3 and 4 of NAK was expressed by Nozick himself (1981, p. 260).

cross-examination takes place. This means that the belief that the witness is reliable might be true but cannot count as knowledge prior to examination, since what we do not have at our disposal is an external method M. An opponent of this view might reply that the witness may have an internal method, e.g. a personal recollection of a past fact, to justify his or her own beliefs. Internalism on epistemic methods is also supported by Nozick (1981, pp. 184–186), who holds an internalist specification of methods, so that two methods are identical if and only if the perceptive data involved in them are the same (even though knowledge is externally grounded). But an internal specification of method should be sound, even though it is rather difficult to establish soundness criteria for internal methods. The sloppy scientist may use an internal method for doing his or her research; nonetheless, such a method does not seem to produce objective knowledge, as science is supposed to do. If it does, this is due merely to epistemic luck; though, the psychological genesis of scientific knowledge should not be confused with its rational, external and objective reconstruction. In order to prevent the use of irrational methods in the analysis of knowledge, Nozick (1981, p. 196) suggests adding to NRAK the condition for which subject S does not believe the negation of 3° and 4°. Yet, also in this case, it is not clear, as observed by Kripke (2011), to what extent such new conditions can prevent problems arising within the irrationality of methods in the theory of knowledge.[10] Kripke moreover noted that, even though the experimental design would include a control group, as long as the experiment was successful, the scientist would satisfy condition 3°, albeit no-one has any reason to believe that it is so. In this case too, no controls *actually* need to be applied, since according to Nozick what is relevant for the analysis of knowledge is merely the internal specification of the *existence* of an external method. Not even the external method is required to be *actually* applied in order to convey knowledge, which may turn out to be problematic.[11]

We have seen that the concept of placebo effect, because of its doxastic specificities, has been used by distinguished philosophers to explicate the interplay between truth and belief and between internist and externist aspects of knowledge. As I point out in the next section, such interplay is also crucial when assessing the meaning of the placebo effect in the clinical context, since higher-order beliefs, particularly sensitive to the clinical context, are involved in the placebo effect.

---

[10] Kripke imagines the following modification of his example: "we may modify the medical case so that the experimenter is even more irrational. Suppose that he has been told many times of the necessity for the use of control groups to exclude the placebo effect, that he has well understood the argument, and that he has acknowledged its cogency. If the experimenter, ignoring what he has learned before, nevertheless irrationally proceeds with his sloppy procedure, none of these additional stipulations prevents Nozick's conditions from being satisfied" (Kripke 2011, p. 172).

[11] The lack of critical reflection on the justification condition for knowledge by Nozick seems to be one of the main sources of the oddities associated with his account of knowledge.

7.4 Placebo Effect and Clinical Reasoning

Beyond clinical research, placebos are routinely used in the clinical context (Hróbjartsson and Norup 2003; Nitzan and Lichtenberg 2004; Louhiala 2012, 2020; Howick, Bishop et al. 2013). Placebos in clinical practice can hardly be said to be curative (Kaptchuk and Miller 2015). Nonetheless, they represent a seminal tool for connecting healing acts in clinical practice with patient's and doctor's beliefs. Although placebo-based beliefs are commonly identified as self-fulfilling, deeper analysis and empirical research on the placebo effect in the clinical setting have emphasised that a patient's mere belief in the improvement of his health conditions does not suffice to justify the occurrence of a placebo effect. As we have already seen, if we ask to the patient P taking the placebo why P feels better, a correct answer of P would be "only because I believe I will get better". This can hardly be considered as an explanation of the phenomenon, and expresses some oddities connected with reasoning about placebo-based beliefs (Smullyan 1987; Cave 2001; Clark 2012). In addition, self-fulfilling beliefs seem to be able to even change evidence. Let us suppose that you have weak evidence that you will pass an examination; however, you know that if you believe you can pass it, this fact would increase your confidence. Conversely, if you are more confident, it is more likely that you pass the exam (Foley 1991).

Let us go back to a medical context. Patients' and doctors' beliefs (of different order) *together with* clinical context (e.g. doctor-patient interaction, medical rituals, etc.) are jointly required if a placebo effect is to take place (Benedetti 2009). The formation of placebo-based beliefs does not occur in isolation but in a multi-agent context. Let us consider the following statement associated with placebo-based beliefs in clinical practice:

(A) "The patient will get better because he believes he will get better".

The doctor believes A, and if the patient also believes A, then the patient's belief in A is a *justification* for doctor's belief in A, while the patient's belief in A is unjustified because it is self-referential (Cave 2009). This is the case when there is a contrast between two agents on what they may reasonably believe: the justification of the belief on one of them depends on the belief of the other. If these conditions are in fact available and I am one of the agents (i.e. the patient), then it is possible to incur in the "placebo paradox", in which it seems that beliefs can be justified (or not) only after having established who the holder of the belief is. My belief is that A is unjustified, whereas the doctor's belief in A may be justified, even though it is based on my unjustified belief in A. It follows that higher-order beliefs are required to justify a belief of a lower level. This is made clear in Lewis' analysis of convention, which also contains precious indications on the issue we are primarily interested in, i.e. self-fulfilling beliefs. Lewis (1975) provides an analysis of convention as a solution to coordination problems. He states that a regularity R is a convention in a population P if and only if, within P, the following conditions hold:

(1) Everyone conforms to R.

(2) Everyone believes that the others conform to R.

(3) This belief that others conform to R gives everyone a good and decisive reason to conform to R itself.

(4) There is general preference for general conformity to R rather than slightly-less-than-general conformity—in particular, rather than conformity by all but any one.

(5) R is not the only possible regularity meeting the last two conditions. There is at least one alternative R' such that the belief that the others conformed to R' would give everyone a good and decisive practical or epistemic reason to conform to R' likewise.

(6) Finally, the various facts listed in conditions (1)–(5) are matters of common (or mutual) knowledge: they are known to everyone; it is known to everyone that they are known to everyone, and so on (Lewis 1969, 1975; see also Chiffi 2012).

According to Lewis, a convention requires at least the contemplation of an alternative regularity R'; otherwise, the convention would be useless. For instance, a regularity R' which implies the administration of no treatment in place of a placebo might give everyone a good and decisive practical or an epistemic reason to conform to R' likewise. Let us focus on the self-fulfilling nature of beliefs. The beliefs of all the members of a population have a self-fulfilling nature when "reasons for conforming to a convention by believing something—like reasons for belief in general—are believed premises tending to confirm the truth of the belief in question." (Lewis 1975, p. 5).[12] Therefore, self-fulfilling beliefs in a multi-agent context require higher-order beliefs working as a justification for lower level beliefs. Moreover, following Lewis' perspective, it is desirable to have common knowledge for these higher order beliefs such that everyone may confirm to R.

In the case of the rituals associated to placebo-beliefs, they do not seem to constitute a *convention* in Lewis' sense, because some conditions are violated. Nonetheless, Lewis' analysis of convention may highlight some specific aspects of placebo beliefs; specifically, it may help us to argue against the self-fulfilling nature of placebo beliefs.

There is no warrant, in the case of placebo beliefs, that both patients and health professionals will conform to a specific regularity R (for instance a clinical ritual). However, if everyone conforms to R and everyone believes that the others conform to R, then conditions (1) and (2) may be justified. According to Lewis' criteria, conforming to a regularity by believing something entails that there are believed premises tending to confirm the truth of the placebo belief in question. As stated before, this issue is related to the self-fulfilling nature of placebo beliefs, which requires, in any case, *both* patients' and health professionals' beliefs. From the point of view of the patient, the belief that health care professionals may provide a good and decisive reason to conform to R is a viable option. The patient believes to receive a non-placebo treatment, and the beliefs of health care professionals may conform to

---

[12]Of course, the analysis of the notions of belief, truth, and knowledge in the placebo effect do not cover all the possible issues related to such phenomenon. However, it sounds reasonable to use the placebo effect only when the epistemic requirements for its existence are fulfilled. One of such aspects, which is quite unexplored, is associated with higher-order beliefs.

a regularity R expressed, for instance, by executing (dummy) clinical rituals. From the point of view of health care professionals, the belief that the patient conforms to R may not count as a decisive reason to conform to R. Unfortunately, there is a great variability at an individual level on the conditions favouring the placebo effect (Benedetti 2009). Of course, if they do, then it follows that clinical rituals and a favourable context *may* contribute to raising the placebo effect. However, there is no certainty that this occurs at an individual level with a specific patient. Lewis requires that the self-fulfilling dimension of these beliefs must be shaped by (i) shared higher-order beliefs providing a possible *ground* for agents' first-order beliefs and (ii) by their conditional preferences. Thus, appropriate higher-order beliefs are necessary in order to have self-fulfilling beliefs in a multi-agent context. This seems not to be the standard situation for placebo beliefs, since patients' and doctors' beliefs do not always share higher-order beliefs.[13] Hence, placebo beliefs are not self-fulfilling in any case: they may lack the appropriate shared ground (among epistemic agents) provided by higher-order beliefs.

Empirical research has in fact confirmed that in the case of a "hidden" administration of a drug (e.g. by means of a machine pumping the drug at defined time intervals, unknown to the patient), the therapeutic effect turns out to be less effective than the one associated with the standard administration of that drug (done by the doctor or nurse). The same effect occurs when a placebo is administered in a similar way (Colloca et al. 2004). This means that the patient does not have higher-order beliefs on the received (dummy) treatment. Hence, the (high-order) beliefs associated with clinical context play a crucial role in conveying the placebo effect, which is in accordance with the idea that "the study of the placebo effect, at its core, is the study of how the context of beliefs shapes brain processes [...] and, ultimately, mental and physical health." (Benedetti et al. 2005, p. 10390).[14] The beliefs about the clinical context are necessary for the placebo effect, by means of the activation of psychological and neurobiological mechanisms (Finnis et al. 2010). In view of this, some philosophical issues regarding the alleged self-fulfilling nature of placebo-based beliefs and their epistemological implications may receive new insights. This is the type of case in which (clinical) evidence may refine philosophers' intuitions and vice versa.[15] If we reconsider NAPB, it is now clear that shared higher-order beliefs

---

[13]It is conjecturable that even in case of open label placebo, patient and doctor do not share all the higher-order beliefs on the placebo treatment.

[14]It is pointed out in (Benedetti et al. 2005) that emotions and individual values too play a non-secondary role on the placebo effect. The main mechanisms associated to the placebo effect are the following three: (i) *classical conditioning*, in which a natural stimulus is repeatedly associated to an unconditioned stimulus, a process that can occur both consciously and unconsciously; (ii) *expectation* (which is always conscious), related to the beliefs and goals of an agent; and (iii) an *affect theory*, in which the key role is played by the appraisals as those cognitive evaluations of problematic situations that can integrate different kinds of information usually required for the conceptualization of personal meanings and expected values (Goli et al. 2016; Ashar et al. 2017). For a new philosophical analysis of placebo effect based on affect theory and the meaning model, see Chiffi et al. (2021).

[15]On the interplay between expert evidence and philosophers' intuitions, see Hitchcock (2012).

between different agents are required. Such beliefs are associated with those mechanisms *activated within a clinical context*. A (dummy) treatment may be administered only in particular circumstances that shape the effect of the therapy; even when a placebo is administered in place of a therapy, the clinical context may contribute to modify patients' beliefs and wellbeing. The clinical context really makes a difference to the placebo effect, since it may change (higher-order) beliefs. This is a nice example of interaction between mind and body and between external and internal aspects of knowledge. The truth of placebo-based beliefs is not something merely internal, i.e. existing in the patient's mind; it is inherently structured on the clinical context which imposes severe constraints on the patient's and doctor's belief formation on the therapeutic value of a treatment. This means that the truth of such beliefs is not unrelated to truths of the external world (specifically, the clinical context), as it is the case for other types of common beliefs.

Let us reconsider NAPB. It does not seem adequate to rearrange the notions of truth and knowledge for placebo-based beliefs, thus violating NAPB1, since it is clinical context which deeply shapes placebo beliefs. But NAPB2 does not hold either, since the truths associated with a placebo effect are not "simply independent of our beliefs"; in fact, the placebo effect cannot occur without personal beliefs of different level on the treatment. In short, the NAPB argument does not seem to capture the complexity of knowledge due to placebo-based beliefs. What is missing in this picture is the clinical context and its interaction with different sources and levels of beliefs that may activate many mechanisms favouring the placebo effect.[16]

7.5   Conclusions

Many problems arise from the notion of placebo. To begin with, a standard definition of placebo and placebo effect is still lacking. The real value of using placebo controls rather than active controls in clinical research is not very clear, whereas the use of the (intuitive notion of) placebo in clinical practice seems to have a remarkable therapeutic significance. What is an ongoing issue is how to assess the nature of the beliefs involved in the placebo effect. Epistemologists have investigated these types of beliefs, which cannot easily be handled by standard theories of knowledge.

Nozick (1981) and Kripke (2011) have used the concepts of placebo and placebo effect in order to clarify the relation between beliefs and truth. Placebo-based beliefs seem *prima facie* to challenge the intuitive notion of truth as correspondence with an external situation. Epistemologists assume placebo-based beliefs to be self-fulfilling, meaning that they become true simply because they are believed as such. I have challenged this view, adopting Lewis' perspective for which self-fulfilling beliefs require higher-order beliefs for their justification and, ideally, common knowledge between different epistemic agents. Such conditions are normally violated in case of

---

[16]However, note that nothing prevents NAPB to be a valid dichotomy for other types of beliefs.

placebo-based beliefs, which in fact can hardly be considered self-fulfilling, since they occur in a multi-agent context.

I have examined Nozick's tracking knowledge theory and analysed Kripke's counterexample to it, which is based on the notion of placebo in a clinical trial lacking proper controls. The Kripkean example has the merit of unravelling the possibility of using irrational methods, which does not seem to be a good property of Nozick's account of propositional knowledge. Then I have analysed the disjunctive argument NAPB. In Nozick's analysis of knowledge, belief-dependent truths seem to require a different account of truth; alternatively, we must base our notion of truth as simply independent of our beliefs. The denial of the self-fulfilling dimension of placebo-based beliefs implies an interplay between both external and internal epistemic factors. I have argued that neither of the options contained in NAPB can make sense of placebo-based beliefs. Such type of belief is analysed by Nozick without taking into account the essential role of higher-order beliefs for different agents.

Lastly, the placebo effect seems to be an ideal field of interdisciplinary research for testing some foundational aspects of the theory of knowledge, and for shedding light on the subtle interplay among beliefs of different levels and sources.

References

Adams, F., Clarke, M.: Resurrecting the tracking theories. Aust. J. Philos. **83**(2), 207–221 (2005)
Ashar, Y.K., Chang, L.J., Wager, T.D.: Brain mechanisms of the placebo effect: an affective appraisal account. Ann. Rev. Clin. Psychol. **13**(1), 73–98 (2017)
Benedetti, F.: Placebo Effects. Understanding the Mechanisms in Health and Disease. Oxford University Press, Oxford (2009)
Benedetti, F., Mayberg, H.S., Wager, T.D., Stohler, C.S., Zubieta, J.K.: Neurobiological mechanisms of the placebo effect. J. Neurosci. **25**(45), 10390–10402 (2005)
Brody, H.: The placebo response: recent research and implications for family medicine. J. Fam. Pract. **49**, 649–654 (2000)
Cave, P.: Too self-fulfilling. Analysis **61**(2), 141–146 (2001)
Cave, P.: This Sentence is False: An Introduction to Philosophical Paradoxes. Continuum, London (2009)
Chiffi, D.: Idiolects and language. Axiomathes **22**(4), 417–432 (2012)
Chiffi, D., Grecucci, A., Pietarinen, A.-V.: Meaning and affect in placebo effect. J. Med. Philos. (2021) (forthcoming)
Clark, M.: Paradoxes from A to Z. Routledge, London, NY (2012)
Clark, P.I., Leaverton, P.E.: Scientific and ethical issues in the use of placebo controls in clinical trials. Annu. Rev. Public Health **15**(1), 19–38 (1994)
Colloca, L., Lopiano, L., Lanotte, M., Benedetti, F.: Overt versus covert treatment for pain, anxiety, and Parkinson's disease. Lancet Neurol. **3**(11), 679–684 (2004)
Comesaña, J.: Knowledge and subjunctive conditionals. Philos. Compass **2**(6), 781–791 (2007)
de Craen, A.J., Roos, P.J., De Vries, A.I., Kleijnen, J.: Effect of colour of drugs: systematic review of perceived effect of drugs and of their effectiveness. BMJ **313**(7072), 1624–1626 (1996)
Finnis, D.G., Kaptchuk, T.J., Miller, F., Benedetti, F.: Placebo effects: biological, clinical and ethical advances. Lancet **375**, 686–695 (2010)
Foley, R.: Evidence and reasons for belief. Analysis **51**(2), 98–102 (1991)
Gettier, E.: Is justified true belief knowledge? Analysis **23**(6), 121–123 (1963)

Giaretta, P.: Modi diversi di concepire l'effetto placebo. Med. Storia **4**, 51–78 (2013)

Goli, F., Rafieian, S., Atarodi, S.: An introduction to the semiotic approach to the placebo responses. In: Goli, F. (ed.) Biosemiotic Medicine, pp. 1–21. Springer, Cham (2016)

Golomb, B.A.: Paradox of placebo effect. Nature **375**(6532), 530 (1995)

Grünbaum, A.: Explication and implications of the placebo concept. In: Andersson, G. (ed.) Rationality in Science and Politics, pp. 131–158. Kluwer, Dordrecht (1984)

Hempel C.G.: Science and human values. In: Aspects of Scientific Explanation and Other Essays in the Philosophy of Science, pp. 81–96. The Free Press, New York (1965)

Hill, A.B.: Medical ethics and controlled trials. BMJ **1**(5337), 1043–1049 (1963)

Hintikka, J.: Knowledge and Belief: An Introduction to the Logic of the Two Notions. Cornell University Press, Ithaca, NY (1962)

Hitchcock, C.: Thought experiments, real experiments, and the expertise objection. Eur. J. Philos. Sci. **2**(2), 205–218 (2012)

Howick, J.: Questioning the methodologic superiority of 'placebo' over 'active' controlled trials. Am. J. Bioeth. **9**(9), 34–48 (2009)

Howick, J.: The Philosophy of Evidence-Based Medicine. BMJ Books/Wiley-Blackwell, Oxford, NY (2011)

Howick, J., Bishop, F.L., Heneghan, C., Wolstenholme, J., Stevens, S., Hobbs, F.D., Lewith, G.: Placebo use in the United Kingdom: results from a national survey of primary care practitioners. PLoS ONE **8**(3), e58247 (2013)

Hróbjartsson, A., Norup, M.: The use of placebo interventions in medical practice—a national questionnaire survey of Danish clinicians. Eval. Health Prof. **26**(2), 153–165 (2003)

Johansson, I., Lynøe, N.: Medicine & Philosophy: A Twenty-First Century Introduction. Ontos Verlag, Frankfurt (2008)

Kaptchuk, T.J., Friedlander, E., Kelley, J.M., Sanchez, M.N., Kokkotou, E., Singer, Kowalczykowski, M., Miller, F.G., Kirsch, I., Lembo, A.J.: Placebos without deception: a randomized controlled trial in irritable bowel syndrome. PLoS ONE **5**(12), e15591 (2010)

Kaptchuk, T.J., Miller, F.G.: Placebo effects in medicine. N. Engl. J. Med. **373**(1), 8–9 (2015)

Kripke, S.A.: Nozick on knowledge. In: Philosophical Troubles: Collected Papers, vol. 1, pp. 162–224. Oxford University Press, Oxford (2011)

Lewis, D.: Convention: A Philosophical Study. Harvard University Press, Cambridge, MA (1969)

Lewis, D.: Language and Languages. In: Gunderson, K. (ed.) Minnesota Studies in the Philosophy of Science, vol. VII, pp. 3–35. University of Minnesota Press, Minneapolis (1975)

Louhiala, P.: What do we really know about the deliberate use of placebos in clinical practice? J. Med. Ethics **38**, 406–407 (2012). https://doi.org/10.1136/medethics-2011-100420

Louhiala, P.: Placebo Effects: The Meaning of Care in Medicine. Springer, Cham (2020)

Luper-Foy, S.: The epistemic predicament: knowledge, Nozickian tracking, and scepticism. Aust. J. Philos. **62**(1), 26–49 (1984)

Makuch, R.W., Johnson, M.F.: Dilemmas in the use of active control groups in clinical research. IRB **11**(1), 1–5 (1989)

Miller, F.G., Brody, H.: Understanding and harnessing placebo effects: clearing away the underbrush. J. Med. Philos. **36**(1), 69–78 (2011)

Moser, P.K.: The Oxford Handbook of Epistemology. Oxford University Press, Oxford (2005)

Nitzan, U., Lichtenberg, P.: Questionnaire survey on use of placebo. BMJ **329**(7472), 944–946 (2004)

Nozick, R.: Philosophical Explanations. Harvard University Press, Cambridge, MA (1981)

Nozick, R.: Invariances: The Structure of the Objective World. Harvard University Press, Cambridge, MA (2001)

Rothman, K.J.: Placebo mania. BMJ **313**(7048), 3–4 (1996)

Smullyan, R.M.: Forever Undecided. A Puzzle Guide to Gödel. Knopf, New York (1987)

Tramèr, M.R., Reynolds, D.J.M., Moore, R.A., McQuay, H.J.: When placebo controlled trials are essential and equivalence trials are inadequate. BMJ **317**(7162), 875–880 (1998)

Worrall, J.: Evidence: philosophy of science meets medicine. J. Eval. Clin. Pract. **16**(2), 356–362 (2010)

Yamada, T.: The epistemic closure principle and the assessment sensitivity of knowledge attributions. In: Rebuschi, M., Batt, M., Heinzmann, G., Lihoreau, F., Musiol, M., Trognon, A. (eds.) Interdisciplinary Works in Logic, Epistemology, Psychology and Linguistics, pp. 181–199. Springer, Heidelberg, New York, Dordrecht, London (2014)

Chapter 8
Nursing Knowledge and the Placebo Effect

8.1 Introduction

Since the turn of the millennium, we have been witnessing new trends in nursing knowledge that are influencing the philosophical and foundational aspects of nursing and clinical practice (Edwards 2001; Tarlier 2005; Risjord 2011; Lipscomb 2012; Thorne 2013; Bluhm 2014). More sophisticated distinctions and argumentations of a philosophically-oriented nursing epistemology are now being integrated classical "nursing theories". The latter were often classified in a 'jungle' of different levels of abstraction such as grand theories, conceptual models, middle-range theories, and so forth. With few exceptions, such levels were based on naive metaphysical and epistemic insights as well as on a misuse of philosophically sound terminology. For instance, when referring to Parse et al. (1985), Johnson (1999) convincingly explained how in Parse's theory there was a confluence of non-sensical and mystical reasoning. Among others, Thorne and Sawatzky (2014) recognized that there still exists an uncritical positivistic ideology in nursing literature.[1] The aim of nursing theories should be not to create an unsound, unclear metaphysical system, but to explore the foundational aspects of the main characteristics of nursing, one of the most important of which is nursing knowledge. This is so because the epistemic nucleus of nursing contributes to defining the distinctive aspects of the discipline. I do not refer to a specific nursing theory; instead, I explore how a philosophical reflection on a particular phenomenon of clinical interest, like the placebo effect, may elucidate some features of nursing knowledge.

---

[1] An uncritical, positivistic attitude, adopting the evidence-based perspective in the clinical context as a dogma is untenable; see (Holmes et al. 2006).

One of the main tasks of the philosophy of nursing today is to analyse nursing knowledge with the philosophical tools of epistemology and value theory, thus shedding new light on theoretical perspectives on nursing. I will first focus on value theory and nursing. In addition to the purely epistemic values associated with (nursing) knowledge (Hempel 1965; Dorato 2004), such as soundness, objectivity and containment of the risk of error (also known as inductive risk), there are other non-epistemic values, such as social, political or ethical values, which have the function of shaping nursing knowledge and of orienting it towards the proper aims of nursing practice. Both types of values are required for a rational reconstruction of nursing knowledge. In particular, non-epistemic values serve the specific purpose of providing guidance on how to apply population-based knowledge to a given context (as appropriate). Nursing theories and models classically accomplished this task, since nursing has been seen as orientated towards the needs of the particular. The different facets of knowing a patient's decisions and beliefs may transcend the biomedical sphere; an aspect that is particularly relevant in nursing (Tanner et al. 1993). In this light, it is usually assumed that a gap exists within nursing between the population-based evidence and the specificities of a particular clinical context. This poses the problem of understanding which model of knowledge translation could take (quantitative) population-based evidence into account, and still be suitable for particular, contingent clinical situations. The relationship between them is not simple. As Thorne et al. (2016, p. 456) put it: "No matter how many cases of a phenomenon one has seen, the commitment to the needs of individuals demands an assumption that each new case may represent new conditions that the nurse is morally obliged to try to discover". This means that the nurse is compelled to discover new hypotheses and possible explanations that may make sense of the uniqueness of an individual in a given clinical context.[2]

In order to explain such a methodological and epistemic gap between the general and the particular, I explore the issue of knowledge translation using a recent methodological framework inspired by the philosophy of science. Consistent with the new methodological trends in nursing philosophy, I provide an example in which epistemological analysis focuses on a specific clinical issue such as the placebo effect. This clinical phenomenon varies considerably from one individual to another, so it is not easy to translate (quantitative) population-based knowledge into knowledge that can be usefully applicable to a particular situation in the context of a "placebo effect". I argue that understanding the main factors associated with the placebo effect in different disciplines is extremely relevant to the analysis of nursing knowledge, which is sensitive to the particular, emerging features of the clinical setting.

---

[2]Nursing knowledge seems to be based inherently on abductive inferences, or in other words on non-deductive inferences intended to find the suitable explanations for clinical phenomena in a given situation. For an analysis of different forms of abduction, see (Magnani 2001). On the role of abduction in nursing, see (Lipscomb 2012).

8.2 Knowledge Translation: From the General to the Particular (and Back)

I focus in this section on two knowledge translation options that may be of some interest to nursing knowledge. The first is the 'cascade' model of science, in which structured scientific knowledge flows from general principles towards practical solutions, thereby becoming evident and manifest. The second is called "emergentism" (Carrier 2010). Emergentists claim that the principles of pure science are not always appropriate when it comes to applying science. It is therefore essential to focus on the practical relevance of theories, rather than on their epistemic principles and values.

The cascade model of science suggests that non-epistemic values may only be associated with applied science in a *contingent manner*, since scientific theories are not necessarily constructed with a definite purpose or for a specific application. From this model, it follows that non-epistemic values may serve only an instrumental purpose: they are needed to arrive at subsequent, more general goals.

Unlike the cascade model, the *emergentist* view thus assumes that non-epistemic values are a key component of scientific knowledge (Adam et al. 2006).

The cascade model foresees a one-way flow from epistemic to non-epistemic values (the applied scientist does not introduce epistemic novelties), whereas emergentism identifies a two-way, interactive relationship between the two kinds of values, allowing new scientific knowledge to arise from applications of science. Such new knowledge may stem from the application of local models designed to handle certain practical situations, which may later require further foundational investigations (Carrier 2004). In any case, it is plausible to assume that no non-epistemic values are inherently associated with the application of science. This means there are no constant, universal or constitutive values of practical relevance in science. There should be a dynamic, epistemic core of theories applicable to different practical contexts. In like manner, practical relevance of nursing knowledge requires no universal criteria of applicability but calls for non-epistemic values capable of orienting its application.

Nursing knowledge consists of an epistemic nucleus in which the methods and findings of nursing theories intersect with other disciplines, thus constituting the grounding needed for nursing intervention. This nucleus may evolve not only from an empirical, but also from a conceptual perspective. Specific non-epistemic values may partially reshape and guide the application of nursing knowledge. It is nonetheless important to point out that nursing knowledge is not like a *turris eburnea*, independent of other disciplines. Nursing knowledge has a professional dimension, which is distinguishable from other types of knowledge mainly in virtue of the crucial role played in it by non-epistemic values.

The problem of particularizing and applying clinical knowledge gained at population level is seminal for clinical reasoning and is far from being a secondary epistemological issue (Giaretta and Chiffi 2013). Complex dialectics and interplay are needed between a knowledge base and nursing practice because knowledge informs practice, and vice versa (Thorne and Sawatzky 2014). As Thorne (2015, p. 6) put it:

"in some instances, a deep exploration of a single case might illuminate something of substantive relevance to the discipline; in others, credibility for our practice audience would be contingent on demonstrating a realistic range of predictable variance". The issue of nursing knowledge translation is therefore a challenging issue from both a clinical and a theoretical perspective.

According to what is now called the emergentist view, "nursing practice is regarded not only as a place of applying knowledge, but also as a place to generate and test ideas for developing knowledge" (Reed 1995, p. 79). This implies that studies should be designed to take possible actions linked to theoretical knowledge into consideration (Thorne 2015). In the next section, I explore the issue of how to set the phenomenon of the placebo effect properly in an emergentist framework for nursing knowledge. I show that the biomedical model, which is basically a cascade model of knowledge translation, is inadequate when it comes to making sense of the main features of the placebo effect.

8.3   The Placebo Effect in Nursing. Beyond the Biomedical Model

Interestingly, the placebo effect stems from a form of clinical knowledge that seems to challenge the cascade model of knowledge translation, in which codified clinical knowledge is merely applied to a specific case. The main limitations of this classical biomedical view relate to the knowledge gained from the placebo effect. In fact, this type of measured response only seems to occur in certain clinical settings, and varies considerably from one person to another (Benedetti 2009).[3] Amongst the classical definitions of placebo and placebo effect, we find the ones given by Grünbaum (1986); according to Grünbaum's poignant definition, placebo is a treatment whose characteristic features do not present any therapeutic impact on a target disease.

Defining placebo and placebo effect is no easy task because, as we have seen, the words commonly used to describe them are "specific" or "inactive", which seems to contrast the fact that a placebo can be an active substance, and also that a placebo effect may be the result of a particular treatment (Miller and Brody 2011). The placebo effect has been studied mainly in medicine, and only a few studies have focused on its relevance to nursing knowledge and practice, e.g. (Connelly 1991; Miller and Miller 2015). I do not intend to provide a new definition of placebo in nursing, but rather to stress the importance of the placebo effect in shaping nursing knowledge. Nursing care is situated in a particular context and inherently associated with the internal sphere of the patient—expectations, beliefs, and intentions—as well as with the external environment (Jarrin 2012). All these factors come into play in

---

[3]Benedetti (2009) pointed out that a *placebo effect* differs from a *placebo-like* effect since the former follows the administration of a placebo, while in the latter no placebo is administered. Still, in both cases, the social, psychological, and clinical background and context around the treatment play a significant role.

the case of the placebo effect. The importance of nursing in enhancing the placebo effect is also shown by the fact that a positive clinical setting can knowingly make a treatment more effective, besides being necessary to favour the very onset of a placebo effect. As pointed out in the second chapter of the book, nursing aims to assess and promote patients' "health potential" vis-à-vis their ongoing state of health (Chiffi and Zanotti 2016). A given patient's health potential indicates the maximal possible enhancement of their quality of life in relation to his or her capacity for self-care. Unlike standard medical treatments, the placebo effect may be a key feature in promoting health in the sphere of nursing. Because of this, the knowledge deriving from the placebo effect may be seen as lying at the very heart of nursing knowledge. Analysing the placebo effect may be a very promising way to understand the *proprium* of nursing knowledge, since this clinical phenomenon is difficult to handle properly from a strictly biomedical perspective, which focuses more on the pathophysiological aspects of a disease than on the patient's perceptions and beliefs. Patients have to be convinced that a (dummy) treatment may be helpful. Such beliefs are usually considered "self-fulfilling" (Cave 2009), i.e. they turn out to be true *simply* by virtue of the fact that people believe them.[4] Strictly speaking, however, merely believing cannot trigger a placebo effect. A positive clinical setting and an interaction between patients and health care professionals are essential too (Benedetti 2009).

Beliefs regarding a placebo do not develop in isolation, but through the interaction with other parties.[5] Administering the placebo, the doctor or nurse believe that the patient will feel better. Let us indicate by "P" the sentence "the patient will feel better". If the patient believes that she will feel better, then the doctor's or nurse's belief in P provides a justification for the patient's belief, expressed by the sentence "I will feel better". Let us indicate by "Q" the sentence "I will feel better". It has been pointed out that there may be good reasons to state that the belief in Q turns out to be unjustified for being theoretically unground, self-referential and paradoxical to a certain extent even when P is justified (Cave 2009). A mismatch between first and third person beliefs may exist. The person who administers the placebo knows about the dummy nature of the treatment, whereas the patient usually does not. Therefore, the patient cannot fully justify the belief in Q, since nurse's or doctor's beliefs are ignored by the patient (Chiffi and Zanotti 2017).

I consider the beliefs responsible for the placebo effect as: (i) *interactive*, because they depend on the relationship between patients and health care professionals; (ii) *situated*, because they occur in a given clinical context related to certain rituals; and (iii) *grounded* on higher-order beliefs concerning what an individual thinks about the beliefs of others. It is therefore essential to know the clinical context and understand other people's beliefs in order to make sense of the placebo effect. As such, we cannot rely on mere population-based information: the placebo effect only works when the (higher-order) beliefs of doctors, nurses and patients interact in a given setting.

---

[4]For a philosophical analysis of this type of belief, also considered in the previous chapter, see (Nozick 1981).

[5]The placebo effect (as well as the placebo-like effect) is not only an epistemic phenomenon because it is also associated with emotional, ethical and ontological factors.

An unsatisfactory clinical context and a patient's negative beliefs may give rise to a nocebo effect, which is the opposite of the placebo effect (Symon et al. 2015). Nurses and other health care professionals often administer placebo substances to their patients (Fässler et al. 2010): they are responsible for creating a favourable clinical atmosphere, and thereby establishing the right conditions for inducing placebo effects and mitigating any nocebo effects.[6] From an ethical point of view, using a placebo in clinical practice would seem to imply deceiving patients (Grace 2006). However, in order to obtain the best health results from a placebo treatment, patients must have untarnished trust for their health care professionals. In fact, it has been reported that even an open-label placebo (i.e. a placebo that is plainly presented to patients as such) may convey a clinical benefit (Kaptchuk et al. 2010). A placebo may be used in clinical practice in accordance with the following ethical directives (Lichtenberg et al., 2004): (i) the intentions of the health professional in using a placebo must be benevolent; (ii) a placebo may be administered when there is the need to alleviate the patient's suffering; (iii) the administration of a placebo must be withdrawn if it turns out to be inefficacious; (iv) a placebo cannot be a substitute for a proven effective treatment; (v) the health care professional must respond honestly if asked by the patient about the nature of the placebo treatment; (vi) if a patient is aided by the administration of a placebo, then it would be unethical to stop its administration.

Nurses are particularly well placed to appreciate the multiplicity of (ethical) factors that can contribute to the onset of a placebo effect. The nurse-patient relationship can strongly influence the placebo effect. This relationship certainly has some non-epistemic consequences, such as the chance to enhance patients' health, but it can be associated with epistemic novelties too. This is particularly true when we consider clinical knowledge based on a person-centred approach to health care (Miles 2009; Miles and Loughlin 2011). Taking this latter perspective, the cascade model of knowledge translation is dismissed in favour of a new model, in which some novel epistemic features of health care can emerge from the doctor-nurse-patient encounter. In this case, there is not just a translation of biomedical knowledge from theory to practice, because nursing knowledge also stems from the psychosocial and humanistic facets of health care. That is why the placebo effect remains an enigma according to the classical biomedical model of knowledge (Pohlman et al. 2013).

Contrary to the view in nursing according to which there would be a need to protect the discipline, or "taking care of the [disciplinary] boundaries to assure survival" (Florczak 2013, p. 314), nursing knowledge does evolve with the epistemological contribution of many sciences, technologies and philosophies oriented towards the non-epistemic specificities and goals of nursing. The fact that disciplines can promote different epistemic and non-epistemic values concurs in blurring the boundaries between them. There is no need to formulate a new nursing theory,

---

[6]The framing of information has been widely studied in psychometric research; this may be important for both placebo and placebo-like effects. It has been observed, for instance, that presenting information in a positive or negative light profoundly influences our intuitive decision-making, and this is particularly relevant in the clinical setting (Tversky and Kahneman 1981).

separate from other sciences, in order to explain the placebo effect. As Risjord (2011, p. 109) argued: "when a scientist draws on a theory that has been confirmed in another domain, she adds the empirical support of that domain to her view. [...] Sharing theory with other disciplines will strengthen nursing knowledge, not dilute it". In fact, the placebo effect is a good example of how the epistemological and scientific dimension (e.g. its biomedical, psychophysiological and philosophical facets) can be fashioned to achieve the distinctive non-epistemic aims of nursing. To maximize patients' health potential, nursing judgments cannot be based on biomedical considerations alone, but must be integrated with nursing expertise and the awareness of patients' preferences. It follows that a nursing approach to properly use the placebo effect should focus on the findings of other disciplines such as psychology, neuroscience, and epistemology, orientating this knowledge towards the specific non-epistemic aims of nursing, which always have an educational flavour whilst promoting independence for the patient's health. To particularize the "general", the patient-nurse interaction is indispensable. Nursing knowledge can be adequately particularized only if new facets of knowledge *emerge* from the clinical encounter with a given patient. This function of nursing knowledge is a hallmark of the discipline. Of course, that is not to say that nursing knowledge should be contextual in every aspect: general aspects associated with knowledge coming from other disciplines can also enrich the formulation and structuring of nursing knowledge. Assuming that new facets of nursing knowledge can emerge in clinical practice, it follows that the knowledge provided by other disciplines cannot be applied without some adjustment. For instance, both nursing knowledge and the placebo effect may contribute to overcoming the classical biomedical model of knowledge translation, in which the analysis of the pathophysiological dimension of the disease may prevail over customized patient care (Miller et al. 2009). This happens in those approaches where clinical knowledge is used and applied by means of nursing diagnoses and interventions with mere taxonomic goals and no clear acknowledgement of the specificity of individual patients.[7] The placebo effect does not fit in with such a taxonomic view of clinical knowledge, since a purely biomedical paradigm tends to ignore the patients' and the health care professionals' beliefs, the clinical context, and the main non-epistemic values of healing acts. In brief, a critical reflection on the use of placebo in nursing may highlight the facets of nursing relating to an emergentist model of knowledge translation, sensitive to a person-centred approach to health care.

---

[7] I have already analysed the taxonomic system present in (NANDA 2012). For this line of criticism on certain taxonomic systems for nursing diagnostics and other taxonomic systems used in nursing, see (Chiffi and Zanotti 2015; Lützén and Tishelman 1996; Pohlman et al. 2013; Zanotti and Chiffi 2015a, b). Suppe and Jacox (1985) proposed to ground nursing taxonomies on conceptual models rather than on inductive generalizations, in order to promote the interplay of concept and theory development that takes place when theories are conformed.

8.4 Conclusion

Two models of knowledge translation have been here presented: the cascade and the emergentist model. While the cascade model refers to the mere application of population-based knowledge to a single case, the emergentist assumes that some epistemic novelties may occur in the interplay between knowledge gained at population level and knowledge instantiated in a single case. Unlike the classical biomedical perspective, in which codified knowledge is applied 'as is' to a given situation, nursing knowledge is more sensitive to the clinical context.

The occurrence of the placebo effect is an example of the patients' participation in clinical practice. The placebo effect may seem to challenge the cascade (or classical biomedical) model of clinical knowledge because it involves patients interacting with health care professionals in a positive therapeutic milieu. Nurses have a special role in inducing placebo effects and containing potential nocebo effects, which is why understanding the placebo effect is fundamental to clinical nursing knowledge. Our investigation, in this sense, delves into some epistemological and clinical aspects of the placebo effect, aiming to show its relevance to the theory and practice of nursing knowledge. As we have seen, the placebo effect is a positive factor that can improve a patient's health. Placebo effects can occur if patients participate in the therapeutic process; and this specific involvement of patients is a distinctive feature of nursing knowledge. By discussing the placebo effect we can clarify some of the many facets of nursing knowledge, and help nurses reflect on how to balance their knowledge gained at population level with the particular, emerging aspects of nursing practice in certain clinical settings.

Finally, the emerging features of the placebo effect in a given clinical context may serve as an example of the so-called "practice-theory gap" (Allmark 1995; Upton 1999), which nurses experience in their daily work. I have explored the epistemological and value-based aspects of this gap, by describing two main models of knowledge translation and the role that epistemic and non-epistemic values play in shaping knowledge. What is still lacking for a thorough understanding of nursing knowledge is an ontological perspective on the nature of the evidence needed to instil a proper grounding for nursing action [for some elements of an ontological view on nursing knowledge translation, see (Doane and Varcoe 2008)]. Future lines of research should therefore focus on the ontological relationships between knowledge translation, evidence, belief formation, and nursing action in the effort to further elucidate the complexity of nursing knowledge and intervention.

References

Adam, M., Carrier, M., Wilholt, T.: How to serve the customer and still be truthful: methodological characteristics of applied research. Sci. Public Policy 33(6), 435–444 (2006)
Allmark, P.: A classical view of the theory-practice gap in nursing. J. Adv. Nurs. 22(1), 18–23 (1995)

Benedetti, F.: Placebo Effects. Understanding the Mechanisms in Health and Disease. Oxford University Press, Oxford (2009)

Bluhm, R.: The (dis) unity of nursing science. Nurs. Philos. **15**(4), 250–260 (2014)

Carrier, M.: Knowledge gain and practical use: models in pure and applied research. In: Gillies, D. (ed.) Laws and Models in Science, pp. 1–17. King's College Publications, London (2004)

Carrier, M.: Theories for use: on the bearing of basic science on practical problems. In: Suárez, M., Dorato, M., Rédei, M. (eds.) EPSA Epistemology and Methodology of Science. Launch of the European Philosophy of Science Association, pp. 23–33. Springer, Dordrecht (2010)

Cave, P.: This Sentence is False: An Introduction to Philosophical Paradoxes. Continuum, London (2009)

Chiffi, D., Zanotti, R.: Medical and nursing diagnoses: a critical comparison. J. Eval. Clin. Pract. **21**(1), 1–6 (2015)

Chiffi, D., Zanotti, R.: Perspectives on clinical possibility: elements of analysis. J. Eval. Clin. Pract. **22**(4), 509–514 (2016)

Chiffi, D., Zanotti, R.: Knowledge and belief in placebo effect. J. Med. Philos. **42**(1), 70–85 (2017)

Connelly, R.J.: Nursing responsibility for the placebo effect. J. Med. Philos. **16**(3), 325–341 (1991)

Doane, G.H., Varcoe, C.: Knowledge translation in everyday nursing: from evidence-based to inquiry-based practice. Adv. Nurs. Sci. **31**(4), 283–295 (2008)

Dorato, M.: Epistemic and non-epistemic values in science. In: Machamer, P.K., Wolters, G. (eds.) Science, Values, and Objectivity, pp. 52–77. University of Pittsburgh Press, Pittsburgh (2004)

Edwards, S.D.: Philosophy of Nursing. An Introduction. Palgrave, New York (2001)

Fässler, M., Meissner, K., Schneider, A., Linde, K.: Frequency and circumstances of placebo use in clinical practice—a systematic review of empirical studies. BMC Med. **8**(1), 15 (2010). https://doi.org/10.1186/1741-7015-8-15

Florczak, K.L.: Protecting the discipline. Collaboration revisited. Nurs. Sci. Quart. **26**(4), 311–315 (2013)

Giaretta, P., Chiffi, D.: Causal attribution and crossing over between probabilities in clinical diagnosis. In: Svennerlind, C., Almäng, J., Ingthorsson, R. (eds.) Johanssonian Investigations Essays in Honour of Ingvar Johansson on his Seventieth Birthday, pp. 191–211. Ontos Verlag, Frankfurt (2013)

Grace, P.J.: The clinical use of placebos: is it ethical? Not when it involves deceiving patients. AJN Am. J. Nurs. **106**(2), 58–61 (2006)

Grünbaum, A.: The placebo concept in medicine and psychiatry. Psychol. Med. **16**(01), 19–38 (1986)

Hempel, C.G.: Science and human values. In: Aspects of Scientific Explanation and other Essays in the Philosophy of Science, pp. 81–96. The Free Press, New York (1965)

Holmes, D., Perron, A., O'Byrne, P.: Evidence, virulence, and the disappearance of nursing knowledge: a critique of the evidence-based dogma. Worldv. Evid. Based Nurs. **3**(3), 95–102 (2006)

Jarrin, O.F.: The integrality of situated caring in nursing and the environment. ANS Adv. Nurs. Sci. **35**(1), 14–24 (2012)

Johnson, M.: Observations on positivism and pseudoscience in qualitative nursing research. J. Adv. Nurs. **30**(1), 67–73 (1999)

Kaptchuk, T.J., Friedlander, E., Kelley, J.M., Sanchez, M.N., Kokkotou, E., Singer, Kowalczykowski, M., Miller, F.G., Kirsch, I., Lembo A.J.: Placebos without deception: a randomized controlled trial in irritable bowel syndrome. PLoS ONE **5**(12), e15591 (2010)

Lichtenberg, P., Heresco-Levy, U., Nitzan, U.: The ethics of the placebo in clinical practice. J Med. Ethics **30**(6), 551–554 (2004)

Lipscomb, M.: Abductive reasoning and qualitative research. Nurs. Philos. **13**(4), 244–256 (2012)

Lützén, K., Tishelman, C.: Nursing diagnosis: a critical analysis of underlying assumptions. Int. J. Nurs. Stud. **2**, 190–200 (1996)

Magnani, L.: Abduction, Reason and Science. Springer, New York (2001)

Miles, A.: On a medicine of the whole person: away from scientistic reductionism and towards the embrace of the complex in clinical practice. J. Eval. Clin. Pract. **15**(6), 941–949 (2009)

Miles, A., Loughlin, M.: Models in the balance: evidence-based medicine versus evidence-informed individualized care. J. Eval. Clin. Pract. **17**(4), 531–536 (2011)

Miller, F.G., Brody, H.: Understanding and harnessing placebo effects: clearing away the underbrush. J. Med. Philos. **36**(1), 69–78 (2011)

Miller, L.R., Miller, F.G.: Understanding placebo effects: Implications for nursing practice. Nurs. Outlook **63**(5), 601–606 (2015)

Miller, F.G., Colloca, L., Kaptchuk, T.J.: The placebo effect: illness and interpersonal healing. Perspect. Biol. Med. **52**(4), 518–539 (2009)

Herdman, T.H. (ed.): NANDA: International Nursing Diagnoses—Definitions and Classification (2012–2014). Wiley-Blackwell, Oxford (2012)

Nozick, R.: Philosophical Explanations. Harvard University Press, Harvard (1981)

Parse, R.R., Coyne, A.B., Smith, M.J.: Nursing Research: Qualitative Methods. Brady, Maryland (1985)

Pohlman, S., Cibulka, N.J., Palmer, J.L., Lorenz, R.A., SmithBattle, L.: The placebo puzzle: examining the discordant space between biomedical science and illness/healing. Nurs. Inq. **20**(1), 71–81 (2013)

Reed, P.G.: A treatise on nursing knowledge development for the 21st century: beyond postmodernism. Adv. Nurs. Sci. **17**(3), 70–84 (1995)

Risjord, M.: Nursing Knowledge: Science, Practice, and Philosophy. Wiley-Blackwell, Oxford (2011)

Suppe, F., Jacox, A.K.: Philosophy of science and the development of nursing theory. Annu. Rev. Nurs. Res. **3**, 241–267 (1985)

Symon, A., Williams, B., Adelasoye, Q.A., Cheyne, H.: Nocebo and the potential harm of 'high risk' labelling: a scoping review. J. Adv. Nurs. **71**(7), 1518–1529 (2015)

Tanner, C.A., Benner, P., Chesla, C., Gordon D.R.: The phenomenology of knowing the patient. Image J. Nurs. Sch. **25**(4), 273–280 (1993).

Tarlier, D.: Mediating the meaning of evidence through epistemological diversity. Nurs. Inq. **12**(2), 126–134 (2005)

Thorne, S.: The evolving nature of nursing ideas. Nurs. Inq. **20**(1), 1–4 (2013)

Thorne, S.: The status and use value of qualitative research findings: new ways to make sense of qualitative work. In: Lipscomb, M. (ed.) Exploring Evidence-Based Practice: Debates and Challenges in Nursing, pp. 151–164. Routledge, London (2015)

Thorne, S., Sawatzky, R.: Particularizing the general: Sustaining theoretical integrity in the context of an evidence-based practice agenda. Adv. Nurs. Sci. **37**(1), 5–18 (2014)

Thorne, S., Stephens, J., Truant, T.: Building qualitative study design using nursing's disciplinary epistemology. J. Adv. Nurs. **72**(2), 451–460 (2016)

Tversky, A., Kahneman, D.: The framing of decisions and the psychology of choice. Science **211**(4481), 453–458 (1981)

Upton, D.J.: How can we achieve evidence-based practice if we have a theory-practice gap in nursing today? J. Adv. Nurs. **29**(3), 549–555 (1999)

Zanotti, R. Chiffi D.: A normative analysis of nursing knowledge. Nurs. Inq. **23**(1), 4–11 (2015a)

Zanotti, R., Chiffi, D.: Diagnostic frameworks and nursing diagnoses: a normative stance. Nurs. Philos. **16**(1), 64–73 (2015b).

Chapter 9
Nursing Knowledge and Values

9.1 Introduction

Values play a key role in the theoretical reflection on science. Recently, as we have seen, a distinction between epistemic and non-epistemic values in science has been assumed (Dorato 2004; Lacey 2005; Elliott and McKaughan 2014). The first are associated with the aims of objectivity, truth and error reduction that all scientific theories must strive to fulfil, while non-epistemic values are intended to guide scientific activity in accordance to some ethical, social or political principles. The importance of epistemic values in science is difficult to refute because of the methodological constrains that are necessarily imposed to any scientific theory; the same does not hold for non-epistemic values, whose role has been often disputed following a positivistic view for which science has to be "value-free", and in particular free from non-epistemic values.

The present analysis shows that epistemic and non-epistemic values have specific roles, which differ from the ones they have in both pure and applied science. Some classical nursing perspectives on nursing knowledge and theory building are critically investigated here from a normative and value-based perspective. The focus will be on the particular nature and the proper aims of nursing: the determination of specific nursing values is used to isolate those features distinctively related to nursing knowledge, which are usually considered difficult to be explicated. Such difficulty derives from a dichotomous perspective on nursing knowledge, which may either refer to the knowledge of a science or an art, without explicitly considering the interaction between these two tendencies (Tarlier 2005). The epistemological and practical consequences of my normative analysis on nursing knowledge may highlight the connection between science and practice in nursing. The aim of the chapter is to defend a perspective on nursing knowledge that is coherent with what is called "moderate emergentist model" of knowledge translation, in which novelties

D. Chiffi, *Clinical Reasoning: Knowledge, Uncertainty, and Values in Health Care*, Studies in Applied Philosophy, Epistemology and Rational Ethics 58, https://doi.org/10.1007/978-3-030-59094-9_9

in the epistemic dimension of nursing theories may come from (but are not directly justified by) the specific aims of its practice. In the previous chapter we focused on the emergentist model and placebo effect in nursing; here I argue that all nursing relevant knowledge may be explained by a perspective of moderate emergentism.

An examination of the nature and of the possible interplay between epistemic and non-epistemic values in science and in different forms of applied science is pointed out in Sect. 9.2. The role of these values for nursing as well as a critical assessment of the nature of nursing are discussed in Sect. 9.3. Concluding remarks regarding the specific aspects of nursing knowledge and values are examined in the final section.

9.2   Epistemic and Non-epistemic Values in Science

Values in science may be characterized as either epistemic or non-epistemic. It is better to say however that values may have epistemic or non-epistemic facets that are sometimes difficult to disambiguate. In the present chapter, I will hold the standard terminology speaking of epistemic and non-epistemic values. Making an analysis of the interplay between the different aspects of values is often a challenging methodological and normative task. In fact, while epistemic values are related to the notions of objectivity, simplicity, effectiveness, etc. (Chiffi and Giaretta 2014), non-epistemic ones involve the ethical, social or political dimension generally associated with scientific work. As opposed to the general consensus about the existence of epistemic values in empirical sciences, attempts at including non-epistemic values in science has not received a favourable response. If we consider science as a mere description of scientific results, then the importance of non-epistemic values might be meagre; but if we also focus on the dynamics of the scientific enterprise, then the need to direct scientific activity towards certain non-epistemic values becomes evident. For instance, all disciplines that aim at promoting health and well-being have to shape their scientific activity towards such non-epistemic values.

As we know, scientific values can also be *contextual* or *constitutive* (Longino 1990; Risjord 2011). Contextual values in science are contingently associated with scientific activity, while constitutive values are those necessary to the scientific enterprise. Note that such distinction regards more specifically the manner in which a normative judgment may change scientific activity.

Contemporary supporters of a value-free science usually state that there is no place for only constitutive non-epistemic values in science, since the epistemic and constitutive value of 'epistemic risk' is unavoidable. Though, if one accepts the existence of non-epistemic values in science, two different versions may be formulated: a weaker one stating that non-epistemic values are merely contextual; and a stronger one affirming that non-epistemic values are also constitutive for scientific activity. An example of the involvement of contextual non-epistemic values in the practice of scientific research can be an engineering scientist engaged in a scientific endeavour with the aim of making money with new patents. At any rate, the legitimacy of constitutive and non-epistemic values in science remains an open issue, essentially because there is no agreement whether they are really necessary for scientific knowledge. The question is thus: is it possible to develop science without including non-epistemic and constitutive values for scientific activity? Let us consider some possible options.

The demarcation between science and non-science is usually based on the notion of empirical (probabilistic) confirmation (Hempel 1952). Simply stated, observational propositions should be empirically testable and inserted into a scientific theory. I briefly outline the classical 'received view' in philosophy of science (based on a cumulative and unsophisticated perspective on scientific knowledge and applications), since it greatly inspired the early formulations of nursing theory. However, contemporary views on the structure of scientific theories in philosophy of science are not so positivistic, but rather geared toward a more fallibilist and pragmatic view on the nature and dynamics of scientific theories.

According to the 'received view' in philosophy of science, a theory should be formalised with a *logical language, formation* and *inference rules, logical* and *specific axioms* as well as *correspondence rules* between some theoretical concepts and observational propositions. Moreover, the theory is usually presented not only with a formal and logically rigorous model but also together with an *intuitive model* (Nagel 1961). For instance, a model of planets rotating around the sun is used as an intuitive model for atomic physics. Thus, intuitive models improve our understanding of scientific phenomena.

Scientific concepts can be seen as the knots of a net representing the scientific theory (Hempel 1952). Though, there is no one-to-one association between concepts and observational propositions, because there is no direct connection between a knot (a concept) and an observational proposition, but rather a path which must be followed throughout a set of knots and an empirical and observational proposition. This means that scientific concepts cannot be reduced to observational propositions. In this classical picture on the logical structure of scientific theories it seems *prima facie* that there is no place for non-epistemic values within the scientific domain.

Independent of the genesis of a scientific theory, a rational reconstruction by means of logical tools and methods is capable of providing a justification of the theory. In this sense, abstracting from contingent features such as its origins, motivations and applications implies that the theory can be justified according to a formal methodology. This implies, as we have seen in previous chapters of this book, that the *context of discovery* must be distinguished from the *context of justification* in which the rational reconstruction of a theory may be provided (Reichenbach 1938). In such a framework, non-epistemic values are not constitutive and may be confined only to the context of discovery of a theory or outside the realm of its justification. Hempel (1965) clarifies however that the justification of non-epistemic values may belong to scientific knowledge when they have an instrumental dimension for achieving intrinsic goals. The validity of instrumental values depends on a more general goal. For instance, Beckstrand (1978) accepts, in the discussion of values in nursing, Hempel's view on instrumental values; she in fact states that the knowledge of instrumental values is scientific knowledge, even if she assumes that the knowledge of what she calls "intrinsic ends" or "goals" of nursing only refers to ethicality, thus reducing non-epistemic values to the ethical ones. As we will see, this is a common feature of many nursing theories.

Summing up the role of values for the 'received view' in philosophy of science, I have thus clarified that non-epistemic values concerning science may: (i) be contingently associated to the genesis of a theory, (ii) be placed at an upper theoretical level since they cannot be directly tested, or (iii) play a role within science as instrumental values.

The notion of applied science can be ambiguous and problematic as well. Applied science may indicate: (i) science in which a well-developed theory or method is used without any revision or extension (for instance, the notion of "applied mathematics"), or (ii) science oriented towards the solution of extra-scientific problems (Hansson 2007). These two senses of "applied science" are not completely equivalent. Yet, for both interpretations it may be argued that the role of non-epistemic values seems to be more important than in pure science, although these can hardly have a constitutive function. It is worth noting that the distinction between pure and applied science is well-defined when we take into account the first sense of "applied science", whereas it may be disputed by the holders of the second illustrated sense. I also hold that there is no loss of epistemic significance for hypotheses in both senses of applied science once the distinction between epistemic and non-epistemic values has been accepted.

The first sense of applied science is similar to what is called the "cascade model of science", for which scientific knowledge flows one-way from general and codified principles towards practical applications becoming evident and manifested. The second sense, instead, is similar to what is called "emergentism" (Carrier 2004), a notion that we have also discussed in the previous chapter in relation to placebo effect in nursing knowledge. Here, I will focus more analytically on the role of emergentism for other facets of nursing practice and knowledge and I will discuss two versions of it. Emergentists claim that the principles of basic science are often unlikely to encounter the demands of applying science. This is why, according to them, it is of primary importance to focus on the practical relevance of theories rather than on their epistemic principles and values. In fact, there is a two-way flow from epistemic and non-epistemic aspects of knowledge. While *moderate emergentists* hold that the goals of practice may partially shape the epistemic components of theories, *strong emergentists* assume that the dynamics of theories may take place independently of any change in the epistemic part of it. I think that a moderate view on scientific emergentism is coherent with the distinction between epistemic and non-epistemic values in applied science. In particular, it explains how practical consequences may suggest epistemic novelties in a theory.

As to the first sense of applied science, it is worth noting that the cascade model refers to a mere application of pure science directed towards a specific goal. Such model of knowledge based on practice is mainly teleologically oriented and shows some similarities with the view expressed in (Wright 1976), which we have already encountered in the second chapter of this book. Wright (1976) stated that the achievement of a goal demands knowledge about the conditions determining the occurrence of an event in the past. If goal A to be reached is causally determined by event B, then in order to make A occur, B (possibly together with other conditions) must be pursued. This approach, called '*consequence-etiology*', is based on the idea of the demonstrated efficacy of an event in the past to achieve a goal in the future. Using Hempel's (1965) terminology, we might say that the judgment of goodness of an action or event is an 'instrumental value' for achieving a goal in the future. As we have seen, Wright (1976) does point out, in fact, that teleological behaviour has a 'consequence-etiology' that is required to bring about some specific goal. Wright's approach seems to be a suitable way to understand the role of non-epistemic values when science is applied as well as, more in general, with regard to teleological behaviour when *codified knowledge* is merely applied to a specific purpose. In the first sense of "applied science" it is clear that there are no constitutive and non-epistemic values, since there are no constant and universal "practical" standards of evidence (Hansson 2007). Following this first sense, values might be considered constitutive with respect to a framework composed by theory *plus* applications. As such, a change in the aims and applications of a theory may entail a change in its (epistemic and non-epistemic) constitutive values, whereas the dynamics of constitutive values are not so regular in science. Hence, the constitutive aspect of values in the first sense of applied science should refer not only to the pure part of the theory, but also to its applications. Indeed, the notion of constitutive value is not used in pure science in exactly the same way as in the first sense of applied science, and the dynamics of epistemic values are not properly justified by this cascade model of knowledge translation.

The emergentist model, instead, refers to the effect of interaction between general principles and practice in shaping scientific knowledge. For instance, when testing whether dioxins have a specific effect or not, an excess of false positives will mean that dioxins seem to cause more harm in animals than they actually do, possibly leading to overregulation of chemicals. Conversely, an excess of false negatives will lead experts to believe that dioxins are less dangerous than they actually are, which may lead to an under-regulation of chemicals (Douglas 2000). It follows that, in applied toxicological research, epistemic values such as 'inductive risk' are associated to non-epistemic values concerning the unnecessary harm imposed on animals or the under-regulation of chemicals. In Douglas' (2000) example, the choice of the level of both statistical errors may have serious non-epistemic consequences. Thus, the choice is made by considering the practical consequences related to specific non-epistemic values. In this sense, non-epistemic values appear to play *prima facie* a constitutive role in applied science when they are related with constitutive epistemic values, as in the case of empirical decisions based on 'inductive risk'. However, there are cases in which epistemic values themselves might be modified in order to make the theory match certain urgent practical situations. Some constitutive and epistemic values in pure theory can, in particular, be adapted to a broader framework for applied science in order to achieve different practice-based goals. In the example made by Cranor (1995), the social costs of adopting standard risk-assessment procedures—currently very slow—for regulating carcinogens are greater than they would be if the regulating agencies provided less accurate but quicker methods. In other words, the non-epistemic value associated to the rapidity of risk assessment seems to deeply influence some epistemic values related to the level of error of the quick, but less accurate methodology. Still, the rapidity of risk assessment is not a constitutive value, and nothing prevents the 'rapid' method from being integrated in the future with the more accurate one. This is why the non-epistemic value of the rapidity of a method does not play a constitutive role for the building of a body of scientific knowledge. Cranor's example, taken from applied science, shows that the adjustment of scientific knowledge to a practical purpose is not an easy task. With that in mind, I prefer a moderate view on emergentism, in which non-epistemic values may only contingently modify the body of scientific knowledge.

So, to recapitulate: for the holders of the cascade model of science, codified knowledge with its epistemic values is merely applied without any modification; yet, there may be cases, as Cranor (1995) points out, in which applied science requires an at least partial adaptation of epistemic values and scientific methods in order to accomplish the pressing social demands of non-epistemic values (e.g. the urgent necessity to test and produce a vaccine for a new lethal disease like COVID-19). My point of view is that non-epistemic values interact with epistemic values, even though they cannot have a constitutive role for (both senses of) applied science, since there are no uniform standards of scientific applications. The safety of a drug can be subject to the practical variability in the application of pharmacological knowledge when, for instance, the safety criteria are examined in normal or in emergency conditions. A distinct body of scientific knowledge with specific epistemic values has to be isolated; and such body of knowledge cannot be *constitutively* modified by the contingency of a specific application. This is required in order to warrant the multi-applicability of scientific knowledge. Still, non-epistemic values can provide an important orientating perspective in applied science, even if they are not deemed to be constitutive of scientific activity.

9.3 Epistemic and Non-epistemic Values in Nursing

Nursing scholars have not always recognized the distinction and interplay between epistemic and non-epistemic (facets of) values. For instance, in a very influential paper, Carper (1978) proposed that nursing knowledge should be examined by means of four patterns, better intended as sources of nursing knowledge rather than types of knowledge (Edwards 2001). The four patterns of 'knowing', viewed as necessary conditions for achieving competence in nursing, are the following:

(1) empirics, the science of nursing, (2) aesthetics, the art of nursing; (3) the component of personal knowledge in nursing; and (4) ethics, the component of moral knowledge in nursing. (Carper 1978, p. 14)

Then, she clarifies that

Nursing [...] depends on the scientific knowledge of human behaviour in health and in illness, the esthetic perception of significant human experiences, a personal understanding of the unique individuality of the self and the capacity to make choices within concrete situations involving particular moral judgments. (Carper 1978, p. 22).

The first and the last patterns are important for our discourse on science and values. We shall not focus on component (2) in which 'aesthetics' for Carper basically means a kind of practical knowledge, nor on the component (3) of 'personal knowledge'. According to the nursing professor, the scientific dimension of knowledge is said to be empirical, factual, descriptive and verifiable, whereas value-laden knowledge for nursing practice is confined to the ethical domain. Thus, in her picture there is no place for epistemic values, nor for the above-mentioned issues about different values in science and their relations. Carper also included knowledge of the goals of nursing in the ethical domain, with the result that the sole non-epistemic values in nursing are the ethical ones. In this framework, normativity seems to be reduced basically to ethicality (i.e. non-epistemic values of a social or political type are not present[1]), and nursing knowledge required for nursing practice ends up being either empirical or ethical.

As we have seen, Dickhoff and James (1968) pointed out a more sophisticated account of nursing theory and knowledge called "practice theory", characterized by severe practical norms and consequences. Starting from the definition of a theory as "a conceptual system or framework invented to some purpose", they claim that four levels with different principles and methods of evaluation can be identified within it. The lowest level is composed of *factor-isolating theories*, which aim at identifying and naming empirical phenomena without imposing any relation among them; in the second level, called *situation-depicting*, empirical phenomena are associated with conceptual relations; while the third level, *situation-relating*, expresses the causal relations among phenomena. These three levels are required to justify a scientific theory; yet, the profession of nursing also requires a fourth level, called *situation-producing theory*, which provides the grounds for creating situations that match the goals of nursing. Dickoff and James clarify that nursing knowledge cannot be value-free, and consequently, normativity cannot be dismissed in the nursing context, since it is a constitutive element of such knowledge. Although Dickoff and James do not explicitly consider the possibility that values may also be epistemic, they believe that there are some constitutive values guiding the aims of nursing activity. Such aims are placed at the top of a hierarchy of theories, whereas the lower levels are based on the causal relations among empirical phenomena. This position in fact matches the 'received view' in philosophy of science, since values may lay on a higher theoretical level than scientific knowledge.

What is fascinating in the position of Dickoff and James is not only the possibility of defining nursing, from a theoretical perspective, as an activity directed towards proper constitutive non-epistemic values and goals, but also the fact that nursing is grounded on scientific knowledge provided by various other disciplines. One thing is clear, though, following this view: if nursing activity must be based on scientific knowledge, then also epistemic values must be incorporated in its body of values.

---

[1]A lack of socio-political aspects of 'knowing' in Carper's picture is pointed out also in (White 1995). However, White's analysis identifies the importance of socio-cultural contexts associated with nursing in the form of situated knowledge, without providing a normative investigation of the specific non-epistemic values of nursing knowledge.

Still, this perspective on nursing knowledge incorporates some features of the cascade model of science. Nursing theories require the first tree levels of empirical and causal knowledge, while non-epistemic values may contribute to select those 'cascades' of empirical knowledge in order to fulfil professional goals. It follows that epistemic components of (the first levels of) theories are not modified by the higher normative level. Non-epistemic values integrate the epistemic ones, but without changing the epistemic nucleus of a theory.

I have pointed out that constitutive non-epistemic values in all senses of applied science show many limitations, which explains why it may be problematic to consider nursing in the strict domain of applied science. This brings us to the question: is it possible to mark a difference in nursing about the use of constitutive non-epistemic values (intended as constant and universal "practical" standards of evidence), unlike what happens in all senses of applied science? If nursing has constitutive values per se—i.e. values existing before the determination of any *specific* application of codified knowledge to practical problems—then it does not behave like an applied science, but rather like a discipline with its own specific principles and goals. Conversely, nursing should also critically use the evidence provided by other sciences and disciplines in order to achieve its goals. The specific values of nursing circumscribe a distinct body of nursing knowledge, which is the result of a critical elaboration of humanistic issues together with scientific and clinical evidence. From this perspective, nursing possesses a distinctive epistemological dimension grounded on specific values, even if such dimension is provided not in isolation, but thanks to the epistemic contribution of other disciplines.

The constitutive non-epistemic values directing nursing activity are usually associated to what are called "conceptual models" (Riehl and Roy 1974), although the terminology is not always uniform in literature. Conceptual models are the reference framework within which more specific and testable theories named "middle-range theories" are built (Fawcett 2012a). These theories have an empirical and therefore fallibilist nature, and they present some epistemic values, such as in the case of "inductive risk". It seems plausible that in a middle-range theory such epistemic values may be possibly adapted, as in Cranor's above-mentioned example, in order to achieve the indications of a specific conceptual model. For this reason, only middle-range theories show some similarities with applied science. Codified nursing knowledge is, in fact, often dynamic since it is "ever-changing with new experiences" (Fawcett 2012b). In some cases, we would probably modify the epistemic values of our middle-range theory in order to match the non-epistemic values provided by a specific conceptual model. But a change in epistemic values is always a very delicate issue, and middle-range theories without conceptual models do not suffice to characterise nursing knowledge. Thus, the nature of conceptual models and the relationship between conceptual models and middle-range theories in nursing represent key epistemological issues. For instance, it has been recently stated, in opposition to Dickoff and James' (1968) hierarchical view on theories, that conceptual models do not represent a kind of upper-level meta-theory, but instead a value-based framework intended to provide an *orientating perspective* for nursing activity (Risjord

2010; Bluhm 2014). In this respect, Henderson's classical position on the proper functions of nursing can be viewed as such an orientating perspective:

> the unique function of the nurse is to assist the individual, sick or well, in the performance of those activities contributing to health or its recovery (or peaceful death) that he would perform unaided if he had the necessary strength, will or knowledge. And to do this in such a way as to help him gain independence as rapidly as possible. (Henderson 1966, p. 15)

This idea of independence in health-related daily activities may be considered a constitutive non-epistemic value for nursing. The role of nursing is thus to respond to self-care needs and at the same time to respect the patient's freedom of choice. What is distinctive about nursing knowledge is its specific aim: its proper function is to evaluate the health 'potential' of an individual, that is, to judge the level of patient independence at a given stage, and to perform interventions based on the evidence—demonstrated effective in the past—in order to restore a future and possibly more independent level of health-related activities. Unlike medicine, in which the main constitutive non-epistemic value is associated with pathological aspects or an alteration from a given norm (Canguilhem 1991), nursing has the proper role of inducing individuals to make the best in order to regulate their psycho-physical processes (Chiffi and Zanotti 2015; Zanotti and Chiffi 2015). It follows that nursing interventions without the patient's active participation are not particularly effective, since the proper non-epistemic values of nursing cannot be fulfilled in such situations. This means that practice in nursing is not a mere application of some codified knowledge: in fact, it results in new knowledge *emerging* from the relation between nurses and patients.[2] Such perspective expresses a *moderate emergentism*, in which some epistemic values of knowledge may be shaped by the purposes of practice. Nursing practice is specifically associated with the non-epistemic value of enhancing the health potential from a more humanistic and social perspective, and not uniquely based on a biomedical and pathophysiological evaluation. Unfortunately, a traditional, medical standpoint that views nursing as an applied science and does not recognise the specificity of nursing knowledge, values and interventions, is still prevailing in the clinical setting (Cody in Daly et al. 1997). Nursing is a practice based on applied sciences, but not an applied science itself because, unlike applied science: (1) it is mainly learned through clinical experience, (2) it aims at particular care rather than uniform production (Bishop and Scudder 1997), and (3) it has constitutive non-epistemic values intended as general "practical" standards of evidence. Notice that Bishop and Scudder (1997) accept (1) and (2), even though they state that nursing has moral values, differently from what occurs in science and art. Indeed, they seem to accept the old distinction between moral and non-moral values, which is often present in

---

[2]This is in line with what has been proposed by Benner et al. (2009, p. 1): "Experienced nurses reach an understanding of a person's experience with an illness, and hence their response to it, not through abstract labeling such as nursing diagnoses, but rather through knowing the particular patient, his typical pattern of responses, his story and the way in which illness has constituted his story, and through advanced clinical knowledge, which is gained from experience with many persons in similar situations. This experientially gained clinical knowledge sensitizes the nurse to possible issues and concerns in particular situations". On the general relation between casuistry and (moral) reasoning, see Jonsen and Toulmin (1988).

nursing literature. The problems with such distinction when applied to the knowledge relative to a discipline are that: (i) moral values are a subset of all possible non-epistemic values, i.e. political or social values are ruled out from such framework; and (ii) non-moral values can be epistemic or non-epistemic, which is too vague. It is also not clear whether moral values have a constitutive or a contextual role in such framework. For these reasons, the distinction between epistemic and non-epistemic values would seem to better characterize nursing knowledge. As a matter of fact, Bishop and Scudder (1997) relied on a dichotomous position that views nursing knowledge as expressing an art or as an applied science, without any overlap and explicit interface between these two tendencies. Yet, it has been shown how nursing knowledge cannot, for instance, derive from a mere scientific evidence-based methodology, but has to take into account the values of *appropriateness* and *feasibility* of nursing interventions (Evans 2003) in order to enhance the health potential of patients. Indeed, my value-based picture implies that nursing is essentially a *practice endeavour with features belonging to both science and art*, in which scientific knowledge guides practice and, in turn, practice shapes knowledge in order to enhance the non-epistemic value of the patient's health potential. This means that nursing is a professional discipline which does not develop independently of the scientific evidence necessary for its practice (Feldman 1981), but which is also integrated and evaluated by nursing non-epistemic values. A critical evaluation of evidence and a calibration or modification of methods of other sciences and disciplines are thus required in order to generate a proper, unique body of nursing knowledge with specific aims. This however does not mean that nursing must simply mimic other disciplines (Cody 1996) because the proper body of nursing knowledge and methods, albeit being enriched by other disciplines, is at any rate *oriented* toward its own specific non-epistemic values.

Summarizing the aforementioned ideas, I have pointed out the prospect of isolating constitutive non-epistemic values and of considering nursing knowledge both as based on scientific evidence and guided by constitutive non-epistemic values.

9.4 Concluding Remarks

The normative and value-based dimension of science has been examined in order to understand the nature of nursing knowledge. I have pointed out the limitations associated with an identification of nursing in each of the two senses of applied science. Applied science may be interpreted as (i) a simple cascade model, in which purely theoretical knowledge flows from general principles to specific applications; or as (ii) an emergentist model where new knowledge derives from practice. I clarified that a *moderate emergentist perspective* is coherent with a distinction between epistemic and non-epistemic values, whereby epistemic values are always associated with empirical sciences. Furthermore, I distinguished values into constitutive or contextual, and provided an example of an epistemic and constitutive value as an 'inductive risk' of error. Then, I considered the limitations of *constitutive non-epistemic* values in science, and underlined that there are no universal "practical" standards in applied science. On the contrary, it has been clarified that the *constitutive non-epistemic value* of nursing is based on the development of individual potentialities in self-care. That in mind, nursing cannot be viewed as (an applied) science nor as an art, but as a *practice endeavour*. The knowledge required for nursing practice is determined by the mutual relationship between its set of scientific evidence and the interpretation of such evidence based on the non-epistemic values of nursing.

The present analysis provides grounds to compare some classical perspectives on nursing knowledge. I have criticized the views on nursing knowledge with which Carper (1978), Beckstrand (1978), Bishop and Scudder (1997) identified non-epistemic values with moral values. I have also focused on Dickoff and James' (1968) position on the nature of nursing theory, who, as opposed to the aforementioned views, did not identify moral values with non-epistemic values; this position is however limited to a view of the cascade model of knowledge translation. I have argued that values in nursing should not be expressed by means of upper-level theories working as abstractions from more testable and empirical theories, which should in fact serve as an *orientation* to nursing practice. In conclusion, I have stated that nursing values are *inherently* required to identify the proper dimension of nursing knowledge, including features that belong to both science and art. In my perspective of *moderate emergentism*, new aspects of nursing knowledge come from nursing practice. Non-epistemic values shape epistemic ones in a constitutive way, and not in a mere contingent way as in applied science.

Future lines of nursing research should focus on how to integrate clinical practice and scientific evidence with the creation of model-based and value-based practice for enhancing the appropriateness of nursing interventions. In this way, nursing should be able to build new explanations through critical and abductive reasoning (Magnani 2001), and to further shape its specific body of knowledge by connecting practice and values.

References

Beckstrand, J.: The notion of a practice theory and the relationship of scientific and ethical knowledge to practice. Res. Nurs. Health **1**(3), 131–136 (1978)

Benner, P., Tanner, C., Chesla, C.: Expertise in Nursing Practice: Caring, Clinical Judgment, and Ethics. Springer, New York (2009)

Bishop, A.H., Scudder, J.R.: Nursing as a practice rather than an art or a science. Nurs. Outlook **45**, 82–85 (1997)

Bluhm, R.L.: The (dis)unity of nursing science. Nurs. Philos. **15**(4), 250–260 (2014)

Canguilhem, G.: The Normal and the Pathological. Zone Books, New York (1991)

Carper B.: Fundamentals patterns of knowing in nursing. ANS: Adv. Nurs. Sci. **1**(1), 13–23 (1978)

Carrier, M.: Knowledge gain and practical use: models in pure and applied research. In: Gillies, D. (ed.) Laws and Models in Science, pp. 1–17. King's College Publications, London (2004)

Chiffi, D., Giaretta, P.: Normative facets of risk. Epistemologia **37**, 217–233 (2014)

Chiffi, D., Zanotti, R.: Medical and nursing diagnoses: a critical comparison. J. Eval. Clin. Pract. **21**(1), 1–6 (2015)

Cody, W.K.: Drowning in eclecticism. Nurs. Sci. Q. **9**(3), 86–88 (1996)

Cranor, C.F.: The social benefits of expedited risk assessments. Risk Anal. **15**(3): 353–58 (1995)

Daly, J., Mitchell, G.J., Toikkanen, T., Millar, B., Zanotti, R., Takahashi, T., et al.: What is nursing science? An international dialogue. Nurs. Sci. Q. **10**, 10–13 (1997)

Dickoff, J., James, P.: A theory of theories: a position paper. Nurs. Res. **17**(3), 197–203 (1968)

Dorato, M.: Epistemic and non-epistemic values in science. In: Machamer, P.K., Wolters, G. (eds.) Science, Values, and Objectivity, pp. 52–77. University of Pittsburgh Press, Pittsburgh (2004)

Douglas, H.: Inductive risk and values in science. Philos. Sci. **67**, 559–579 (2000)

Edwards, S.D.: Philosophy of Nursing. An Introduction. Palgrave, New York (2001)

Elliott, K.C., McKaughan, D.G.: Nonepistemic values and the multiple goals of science. Phil. Sci. **81**(1), 1–21 (2014)

Evans, D.: Hierarchy of evidence: a framework for ranking evidence evaluating healthcare interventions. J. Clin. Nurs. **12**, 77–84 (2003)

Fawcett, J.: Thoughts on concept analysis: multiple approaches, one result. Nurs. Sci. Q. **25**(3), 285–287 (2012a)

Fawcett, J.: Thoughts about nursing science and nursing sciencing on the event of the 25th anniversary of nursing science quarterly. Nurs. Sci. Q. **25**(1), 111–113 (2012b)

Feldman, H.R.: A science of nursing—To be or not to be? Image. J. Nurs. Scholarship **13**(3): 63–66 (1981)

Hansson, S.O.: Values in pure and applied science. Found. Sci. **12**, 257–268 (2007)

Hempel, C.G.: Fundamentals of concept formation in empirical science. International of Encyclopedia Unified Science, Vol. II. No. 7. University of Chicago Press, Chicago (1952)

Hempel, C.G.: Science and human values. In: Aspects of Scientific Explanation and other Essays in the Philosophy of Science, pp. 81–96. The Free Press, New York (1965)

Henderson, V.: The Nature of Nursing. The Macmillian Company, New York (1966)

Jonsen, A.R., Toulmin, S.: The Abuse of Casuistry: A History of Moral Reasoning. University of California Press, Berkeley (1988)

Lacey, H.: Values and Objectivity in Science: The Current Controversy About Transgenic crops. Lexington, Lanham, MD (2005)

Longino, H.: Science as Social Knowledge: Values and Objectivity in Scientific Inquiry. Princeton University Press, Princeton (1990)

Magnani, L.: Epistemic mediators and model-based discovery in science. In: Magnani, L., Nersessian, N.J. (eds.) Model-Based Reasoning: Science, Technology, Values, pp. 305–329. Kluwer Academic/Plenum, New York (2001)

Nagel, E.: The Structure of Science. Hackett, Indianapolis (1961)

Reichenbach, H.: On probability and induction. Philos. Sci. **5**(1), 21–45 (1938)

Riehl, J.P., Roy, S.C. (eds.): Conceptual Models for Nursing Practice. Crofts, New York (1974)

Risjord, M.: Nursing Knowledge. Science, Practice, and Philosophy. Wiley-Blackwell, Oxford (2010)

Risjord, M.: Nursing science. In: Gifford, F. (ed.) Handbook of the Philosophy of Science, Volume 16: Philosophy of Medicine, pp. 489–522. Elsevier BV, Amsterdam (2011)

Tarlier, D.: Mediating the meaning of evidence through epistemological diversity. Nurs. Inquiry **12**(2), 126–134 (2005)

White, J.: Patterns of knowing: review, critique, and update. Adv. Nurs. Sci. **17**, 73–86 (1995)

Wrigh, L.: Teleological explanations. An etiological analysis of goals and functions. University of California Press, Berkeley (1976)sa

Zanotti, R., Chiffi, D.: Diagnostic frameworks and nursing diagnoses: a normative stance. Nurs. Philos. **16**(1), 64–73 (2015)

Chapter 10
Clinical Equipoise and Moral Leeway

10.1 Introduction

Physicians have knowingly the moral duty to offer their patients optimal care. Yet, this deontological obligation does not in all respects conform to the ethics and methodology we find in the practice of clinical research (Miller and Brody 2007). For example, when a physician-researcher informs patients of the possibility to enter a newly-designed Randomized Controlled Trial (RCT),[1] at least two issues have to be weighed upon: on the one hand, a group of randomly-selected patients may be allocated to the control arm of a placebo trial in which the new treatment to be tested might show some efficacy; on the other hand, another group of randomly-selected patients may be allocated to the new treatment arm in which the effect of the given treatment might be some, null or even negative: it can be beneficial, futile or harmful, and to varying degrees.

In this sense, we can see how the ethical principles in clinical practice and those in clinical research do not perfectly match. For instance, in virtue of research-based reasons including curiosity, learning and education, the attempts in confirmatory Phase-III to generalize the validity of the therapeutic protocols over the target population—i.e. those who are, could be or will be in the need of new therapies—might incorporate non-beneficial procedures that impose unforeseen risks to the patients.

A classical solution to the potential conflict between the ethics of clinical research and that of clinical practice is the *Principle of Equipoise*. Such principle is an attempt to define a systematic relation between uncertainty and the moral leeway of conducting an RCT. In brief, it proposes to correlate a change in the level of

---

[1] An RCT is an experiment in which people are randomly allocated to receive one of several clinical interventions. One of these interventions is the standard of comparison or control: the control may be a standard practice or a placebo.

D. Chiffi, *Clinical Reasoning: Knowledge, Uncertainty, and Values in Health Care*,
Studies in Applied Philosophy, Epistemology and Rational Ethics 58,
https://doi.org/10.1007/978-3-030-59094-9_10

uncertainty associated with clinical options with a change in the set of possible actions that are morally permitted.

Yet, for reasons which I briefly review below, the principle of equipoise has come to be rejected in the literature as a "sacred dogma" (Miller 2012). At the same time, many authors continue to defend it and its many variations as valid principles to be adhered to in clinical research.

Different forms of equipoise are available. *Individual Equipoise* (IE) (also, and perhaps unhappily, known as the "theoretical equipoise") is intended to refer to a state of genuine or ideal uncertainty on the part of the clinical investigator regarding the therapeutic value of each of the arms in a clinical trial (Fried 1974). The state of IE is disturbed when the researcher comes to believe (or, in a slightly weaker sense, conjectures) that one or more of the arms of a trial is in fact more effective than the others. In this case, according to IE, early stopping rules are recommended, and the trial is likely to be terminated.[2]

IE is considered to be a fragile notion and easily disturbed in practice. Reasons are at least five-fold: (i) IE is idiosyncratic, as it is adopted in vastly different ways across diverse institutional contexts and cultures; (ii) it is no longer consistent with contemporary and emerging practices in the methodology of RCTs; (iii) it takes beliefs, preferences and conjectures as point-estimates but omits assessing the role of uncertainty involved in the formation of such beliefs, preferences and conjectures[3]; (iv) it is disturbed as soon as new evidence appears to favour one arm of the trial, possibly very early and prematurely in the conduct of the trial in question[4]; (v) it is not conceptually clear how IE differs from CE (clinical equipoise, see below) in its interpretation of what 'a single investigator' means. Perhaps a team carrying out the same experiment could also be conceived as a singular entity, but can it be assumed that the same type and amount of uncertainty is distributed equally among all its members?

It is also worth noting that the initial evidence for a proposed new treatment arm of a trial may be severely weak and subject to various biases affecting the design, conduct and implementation of the trial. As a consequence, it is quite likely that new evidence, which may be incomplete or skewed, fails to yield compelling indications and remains insufficient to change clinicians' beliefs regarding the comparative therapeutic value of that arm of a trial.

Freedman (1987a) has proposed to overcome these methodological limitations of IE by replacing it with the principle of *Clinical Equipoise* (CE), also but not exactly equivalently known as a "community equipoise". Unlike IE, which is related to the states of genuine uncertainty of a *single* clinical researcher or entity, CE states that a trial is not ethically justified if there is "no *consensus* within the expert clinical

---

[2]Stanev (2015) shows that the current practice in adopting early stopping rules may be due to mistaken interpretations of the relevant statistical results, which have their roots in uncritical acceptance of error statistics underlying the decisions to implement these rules.

[3]In the light of this issue, IE might be better expressed using alternative methods, such as confidence intervals or non-additive probabilities, rather than standard probability measures.

[4]These problems are discussed in detail in (Freedman 1987) and (Sackett 2000).

community—not necessarily on the part of the individual investigator—about the comparative merits of the alternatives to be tested" (Freedman 1987a, p. 145).[5] Freedman takes CE to be *necessary* in *all* cases of clinical research, and therefore to be applicable also with study designs that are markedly different from the RCT designs. My purpose in the present chapter is to point out that this wider interpretation of the scope of CE leads to a thesis that may bring about serious epistemological problems concerning the characteristics of the ethical situations one faces in clinical research.

When is CE disturbed? Simply put, CE is disturbed when, in the presence of a known and efficacious treatment A as well as a new treatment B, the evidence gathered in favour of B is so unequivocal that "the committee of investigators believe no open-mind clinician, informed of the results, *would* still favour A" (Freedman 1987a, p. 144). As is the case with IE, this definition of CE faces some inevitable limitations. Initial problems concern the determination of who the experts/investigators are. Does CE concern only physicians, or are also other participants involved in the conduct and oversight of the proposed research such as nurses, administrators, policy makers, public health officials and regulatory agencies, bioethicists and other relevant decision makers? (Veach 2007). How do we ascertain a fair accommodation of a patient's autonomy requirement concerning the freedom of choice of therapeutic options and the CE? (Karlawish and Lantos 1997; London 2007). How do we deal with the scales of judgments present in the expert clinical community, ranging from plausible to unjustified and incorrect?[6] What do we actually mean by an open-minded clinician? And finally, after all these issues have somehow been addressed, a further question still lingers: why is it that in certain situations 'non-open-minded' clinicians could not be more right than others? The emerging distinction from the application of CE between two types of experts suggests that the experts come to the belief that the comparative uncertainty, indifference, and ignorance of therapeutic alternatives are relative to the standards of justification of clinical knowledge. If CE is taken as a decision rule in clinical ethics, then the ethical justification of CE is substantially affected by the epistemological issues concerning the standards of acceptability of clinical knowledge.

For these reasons, I feel that a fresh epistemological analysis of the beliefs involved in judgments of equipoise might help to elucidate some of the key issues everyone is faced with in clinical ethics. Next, in Sect. 10.2. I critically discuss some of the key problems of CE. In Sect. 10.3. I propose that a modification of the methodological principle of hypothetical retrospection (HR) could meet these problems. I argue that,

---

[5]Freedman (1987b) clarified that, beyond scientific validity, an important requirement for medical ethics is the clinical value of a hypothesis. It is specifically on the clinical value that there may be disagreement in the community of experts as indicated by CE.

[6]For a classical analysis of bounded rationality in which the rationality of decisions is shaped by the limitations of time, information and other contextual factors see, for instance, Tversky and Kahneman (1981). Their view, which is "heuristics as errors" in reasoning, takes optimal and analytic procedures to be supplanted in human economizing decisions by suboptimal but fast procedures of reasoning that achieve practical goals with less expenditure on time, money and cognitive effort. For a critical analysis of this paradigm, see (Gigerenzer et al. 1991), among others.

as soon as the underlying and questionable probabilistic assumptions involved both in current interpretations of CE and in the methodology of HR are exposed, we will be able to put the complex interaction between uncertainty and moral leeway in clinical decision making under a clearer light. Section 10.4 concludes the chapter.

10.2   Clinical Equipoise and Its Fundamental Problems

In this section I discuss some critical aspects associated with CE. Most of these aspects have already been discussed in the literature, and various interpretations of CE have commonly been adjoined with proposals of how to solve the problems emerging from them.

Let us first briefly review some of the reactions to these problems, keeping an eye on the epistemological complexities of the notion. One problematic aspect in the definition of CE comes from the collapse between judgments of *clinical agnosticism* and those of *clinical conflicts* (London 2007). Clinical agnosticism would be present when a medical community has no well-defined judgments that could be passed on concerning the relative therapeutic values of the treatment under investigation. The absence of such judgments is commonly due to the lack of quantified and well-interpreted data, negative or failed experiments, inadequate effect sizes, inadequate or flawed statistical calculations, or any combination of these factors. The absence or insufficiency of quantified data may follow from the inapplicability of standard probabilistic methods to the available data rather than from the absence of the data itself. Such inapplicability may in turn be the result of difficulties, or an outright impossibility of calculating the probability distributions of a certain phenomenon. When the former is the case, we would be facing fundamental uncertainty (the presence of *unknown unknowns*) rather than being conditioned on the risks (or *known unknowns*), because only the latter case presupposes that there are probabilistic uncertainties in which conditional probabilistic judgments can be formulated (Knight 1921).[7] Clinical agnosticism, in contrast, suggests the presence of fundamental uncertainty. The difference is that, under the conditions of risk, clinical conflicts are not only possible but unavoidable. Only in the case of the presence of risks can a group of clinicians genuinely disagree or agree-to-disagree with another group on the relative therapeutic merits (or demerits) of a treatment over another. Both groups have some specific probabilistic judgments, which they have received from independent sources and which they can present to support their respective judgments. But when the majority of judgments are in fact grounded on ill-defined or a combination of ill-defined and under-defined values, it becomes much harder to see how a genuine disagreement could arise among them.

In brief, clinical conflict means comparative indifference among potential therapies, in the sense that clinicians can pass on fairly determinate probabilistic judgments

---

[7]The confusion between "conditions of risk" and "conditions of severe uncertainty" is called "Tuxedo Fallacy" (see e.g. Hansson 2009).

of indifference among them. At the same time, usually a minority of clinicians would disagree on those judgments.

In other words, grounds for clinical disagreement should not be confused with genuine uncertainty that prevails among clinical factions. Consider a hypothetical situation in which the entire clinical community agreed on the therapeutic merits of a treatment with respect to some known alternatives, and that all clinicians were at an indifference point: in this case there is both CE and IE. Gifford has observed that in such situations "an arbitrarily small amount of evidence in favour of a treatment A at the beginning of the trial would tip each of them out of equipoise, and the CE criterion would imply that we have collected all the information we needed for approving, for instance a new drug" (Gifford 2007, p. 146). Gifford concludes that this "is surely wrong" and observes that we are looking for *reliable* and suggestive evidence, whatever it may be, and not for evidence that is meant to reach unanimous expert consensus. Gifford imagines a second scenario in which clinicians are all biased: in this case even a *scintilla* of new evidence, which might soon be overridden, might tip them out of CE. This does not seem methodologically correct even in the cases where initial evidence remains unreliable, because also in those cases the principle of CE fails.

Miller and Weijer (2003, p. 100) have clarified Freedman's position by taking trials to "be continued until the evidence gathered is sufficient to resolve significant disagreement within the expert clinical community" (see also London 2006).[8] Initial evidence may not accomplish this task, since such evidence is weak and is likely to have higher degrees of unreliability and error than later evidence obtained from trials conducted for longer periods of time. It is not clear, however, what relative therapeutic merits a suspension of judgment has when judgments are kept on hold until all significant disagreements have been correctly resolved. No scientific experiment is really a decisive, crucial experiment. A good experiment can refute some of the earlier views, and with cleverly crafted hypotheses it can expedite the inquiry that otherwise would have taken much longer; but it typically could not (and in fact should not) be designed or conducted with any consensus-seeking purposes in mind, as that motivation would taint the design and increase the false discovery rate of the trials.[9]

A further but related objection to the widening of the scope of CE taking economical aspects of research into account is that clinical evidence for new treatments

---

[8]Even such continued and completed trials are unlikely to achieve the desired sufficiency of evidence, or evidence that is stronger than the initial evidence from early phases of a trial. Such a phenomenon adds to the reasons why systematic reviews and meta-analyses are also required in order for a research to achieve the evidential status concerning it effect sizes and the respective clinical conditions, hospital practices and proposed treatments. The well-known demand for meta-analyses is due to the problems of amalgamation of different sources of evidence and to the persistent lack of replicability of findings on specific clinical questions. This, in turn, is a symptom of underlying biases involved at all stages of experimentation and publication of results (Ioannidis 2005).

[9]In a similar situation, the designs would be biased towards a likelihood that the effect sizes of trials conducted between competing research teams that work on the same problem are exaggerated by those who are the first to report their positive findings. This is an instance of the bias known as "Winner's Curse".

that seek regulatory approval also requires the pre-clinical Phase I and Phase II studies. This requirement is present even for those early trials that evaluate surrogate rather than clinically relevant endpoints. Acknowledging the problematic association between surrogate endpoints and clinical indications means that early evidence may only loosely justify clinicians' beliefs on the efficacy of the therapies in question (Miller 2011).

However, it would be hasty to conclude that the ultimate reliability of evidence is due only to a proper carrying out of Phase-III RCTs: for one thing, studies with alternative designs can also provide reliable evidence strong enough to ground correct ethical decisions (Worrall 2008; Bluhm 2010). Yet, it should be recognized that the use of surrogate endpoints is usually not considered sufficient to resolve strong clinical uncertainties. At the same time, industry-funded studies tend to take liberties on choosing certain endpoints driven by their own agendas. This poses additional problems for gaining critical overviews and for reliable meta-analyses to be achieved concerning the effect sizes of a significant set of studies that have been or are in the process of being performed. Moreover, at the confirmatory Phase-III stage the new treatment seems to have already (at least *prima facie*) a therapeutic effect *by definition*, and therefore using that fact as a criterion for judgments on the ultimate reliability of evidence in terms of statistical significance rate may be moot.

There is another but related aspect involved in acceptance of the principle of CE. As mentioned in a previous chapter, the use of placebos in clinical research may be problematic, also because these treatments have been likened to deception in clinical practice (see e.g. Annoni and Miller 2014). If CE is assumed to hold—and when an already known active treatment exists—testing new treatments against a placebo arm would lack methodological and clinical value. On the other hand, short-term trials with placebo-controls that evaluate only mild conditions with negligible risks would be (at least in line of principle) ruled out. This does not appear to be a desirable outcome.

It is worth noting that '*active*' *controlled trials* face comparable questions and challenges as well. Among them I list the following three that I already partially discussed in previous chapters but are useful to recall in relation to CE: (1) no adequate, golden standard of reference may exist; (2) no guarantee that an 'active' treatment is invariably effective may exist (or it may well fail under new experimental conditions); (3) the confidence intervals of the new treatment A and the interval of the 'active' control B may overlap. But it is only after one has introduced another placebo arm that we would be prompted to begin to understand whether all three confidence intervals overlap. Thus, there is no difference between the arms A and B with respect to the placebo arm or otherwise (Chiffi and Zanotti 2017). As we have seen, if we add that the terms usually associated with placebo (such as being "non-specific", "inert" or "vacuous") and the distinction between "active" and "non-active" treatments are likely to be misleading (Howich 2011), then every *ex ante* prohibition based on CE to conduct placebo trials rather than active control trials shows several limitations.

The principle of CE has been suggested to serve as an interface between the ethics of clinical research and the ethics of clinical practice. However, it is important to recognize that many connections between these two areas of activity do *not* appear to be associated with principles like CE or its variants. For example, the investigator has the specific moral duty of non-exploitation of the patients (Miller and Brody 2007): this obligation carries over to situations in which research-driven goals and the aims of the clinical practice are far from being tantamount. A clear example of a conflict between the physician's responsibility for the care of a patient and the responsibility for the internal validity of an RCT was provided by Sackett (2000), who personally acknowledged a conflict in his own responsibility for the care of one of his patients with the validity of an RCT. Yet, other authors believe that a fiduciary obligation among patients and doctors (Miller and Weijer 2006) override the principle of non-exploitation.

Aside from the principle of non-exploitation (or fiduciary obligation) and the possible exclusion of CE, other principles are clearly required to ascertain the ethical conduct of clinical research, such as fair subject selection, informed consent and scientific validity (Emanuel et al. 2000). When all these principles are taken into account, the various uncertainties involved are no longer negligible.

10.3 Uncertainty and Moral Leeway

From a general perspective, CE is an attempt to systematically relate different forms of uncertainty with the moral leeway faced in clinical decision-making and practice. In argumentation theory, there exists a new and promising approach, called *hypothetical retrospection* (HR), which has been developed to deal with judgments of uncertainty and moral permissibility (Hansson 2007). This approach takes values regarding decisions to be evaluated under the assumption that certain future scenarios have readily materialized. The evaluation of actions is nevertheless performed considering both values and evidence that were available in the past, *at the moment of the decision*. The criterion for the decision rule to apply assumes that retrospective judgments yield a scenario, which turns out to be ethically acceptable from *all* such hypothetical retrospections.

Applied to the conduct of RCTs, this means that already the study design phase would narrate a range of hypothetical future situations that would or could emerge from the various arms of the trial, while some others may be ruled out. In fact, the moral status of the actions of the present is evaluated precisely from the angle taken by these hypothetical situations, *with the knowledge that is being obtained at the present moment.*

To hypothesise retrospectively means that we are able to imagine a range of future scenarios that could plausibly materialize from the actions that we choose to perform today. We are thus asked to put ourselves into those scenarios, one by one. Having done this imaginative 'time-travel', we are invited to look back and reflect on those decision points, while being asked: is your current scenario an acceptable, or even a desirable one, that came about as a result of that earlier decision? You are then to collect all those scenarios that emerge as acceptable or desirable and to conclude that ethically acceptable decisions were all those that led you to those hypothetical situations from which you were able to reflect back in time and which you had found desirable.

The epistemic condition involved here is that, when you travel into the future, your epistemic state does not change; when you live in those hypothetical scenarios you are not allowed to know anything more than what you knew when the relevant decision points were obtained. For example, you do not know, inside that future scenario, whether the effect sizes were in fact true, or whether the proposed experimental therapy was in fact more efficacious than another one, or finally which future facts had intervened during the process. You are not supposed to know, in general, what the relevant future findings of science and evidence-based medicine might have been, or what the post-hoc alternatives could have possibly been.[10]

Imagine what the application of such a method of hypothetical retrospection could mean from the points of view of a patient. Suppose that a patient seeks, say, to enrol in a Phase-II clinical trial that concerns an experimental therapy for some previously incurable disease. The desirable scenarios are surely those in which a progression-free state of the disease obtains, or even its remission, while the outcomes that contribute to the diminished prognostics such as relapses and refractory responses would be ruled out.[11] Since none of these scenarios are by any means determined by the current state-of-the-art of the conduct of the trial in question, and since they cannot be taken to be strictly causal consequences of certain pharmacological and physiological facts of the therapy, their value lies primarily in having been produced as narrations that aid the decision-making deliberations of the present time.

These retrospections are thus not intended to answer whether the proposed therapies also work for *us*; they are intended to address the question of understanding the condtions for their plausibility. The lesson of this approach is that, if the design of RCTs could take into consideration a decent range of those narrations, it might become possible to think of the ethical values involved in scientific, translational and clinical research and practice in a somewhat wider perspective than before.

In this sense, HR appears to me as a promising alternative to think about the moral permissibility of a large variety of actions and their ethical value, among which some difficult and previously unanswerable decisions involved in clinical research and practice. However, given its rather complex and unconventional logical structure, the method of HR might never become a widely popular mode of reasoning. In fact, HR is not without problems either. In order to improve the methodology as well as to widen the scope of its applicability, I identify one particular problem in one of its assumptions. And in the course of doing so, another problem comes to the fore that undermines the validity of using CE as a crucial criterium for resolving clinical conflicts that involve the consideration of moral values. A wider upshot is that we might get a revised form of HR that is better adapted for the context of medical and clinical decision-making and which could, in fact, become a new way of thinking about moral decisions influenced by fundamental uncertainty.

---

[10]The logical model for such hypothetical retrospections is a branching-time model.

[11]*Exitus* may or may not be ruled out, depending on the patients' desires, wishes, wills and testimonies, severity of conditions and the gravity of suffering, among other factors.

What I want to focus on next is a particular aspect of the methodology of HR. HR contains a principle (or a general tendency to act), which has been taken to regulate its methodology, called *uncertainty transduction* (UT). UT states that "uncertainty widens the range of acceptable, or morally permitted, alternatives that are open" (Hansson 2007, p. 153). As far as CE is concerned, for example, we find a certain form of such uncertainty transduction in the following case: a change in the level of uncertainty in clinical research typically entitles one to argue for both the moral *and* scientific permissibility of a new trial.

Yet UT is problematic in a similar sense in which CE is. My view in fact is that the purpose of UT has been (to a sufficient degree) the same as the purpose of CE: both principles look for an *ex ante* method that would systematically connect uncertainty to permissible actions. To put this bottom-line into the perspective of a case, it is possible to consider the following example, which comes from Hansson (2007): a husband surprises his wife by buying two cinema tickets for her birthday. There are only two plays to attend. If the husband is aware of which play his wife prefers, he would feel obliged to buy the ticket for that specific play; however, if he is uncertain about his wife's preferences, he may feel free to buy the ticket for the play that he himself prefers.

The greater the uncertainty, the greater the range of acceptable actions for the husband—or so it seems. This intuitive notion is nevertheless deceptive. Counterexamples to UT can easily be formulated as follows: a pharmaceutical company has the choice of entering the market with two drugs, A and B. They do not differ in production price or efficacy, and the choice depends only on two factors both potentially harmful to health: immunosuppression and cytotoxicity. There are two scenarios to consider. In Scenario 1 it is known that A is more suppressive than B, while nothing is known about the toxicity of the products. In Scenario 2 it is known that A is more suppressive than B but, in this case, toxicity data are available showing that B is moderately toxic, whereas there is no indication of the toxicity for product A (cf. Hansson 2013). While the first scenario is coherent with UT, the second makes it plausible to choose indifferently among one of the two options, which would be contrary to what UT proposes. In the first example, there is the implicit assumption that no further scenarios are real alternatives to the two proposed scenarios; in the second, instead, it may be plausible to assume that some new scenarios, in addition to the proposed ones, may arise, which would indicate, for instance, some toxicological information on the substance A. We can see from this example that the way we give structure to future scenarios does affect our present choices. Further counterexamples that undermine the validity of UT have been presented in the recent literature.[12]

But when we are dealing with severe forms of uncertainty, what are the proper structures of future scenarios? Djulbegovic (2007) has proposed that alternate futures accommodate the uncertainty associated with RCTs, and that the alternate structure

---

[12]Common examples of the failure of UT can be drawn from game theory. Let us mention two: (1) games that use the "burning bridges" strategies involve actions that intentionally limit the range of one's own options in order to signal a credible commitment to the opponent as well as the way to avoid a conflict; and (2) games in which the epistemic states of the agents are also taken into account in the decisions (see Chiffi and Pietarinen 2017).

is the form of future assumed in CE. Yet, even though this view may be plausible for some types of RCTs,[13] the perspective of alternate futures is problematic when it concerns novel, innovative and future RCTs rather than only regulatory and confirmatory ones: it becomes restrictive to assume that every time we conduct an RCT we would face a finite set of future scenarios with certain well-defined alternatives (even if with possibly uncertain outcomes). Moreover, the very case in which RCTs are designed to involve considerations of alternative futures may be solely due to the tendencies to safeguard termination of those trials (Broderick 2013). Still, scenarios that follow from safety data would hardly cover more than the formal part of the larger story of alternative futures. After all, RCTs can provide only a limited amount of safety data, since the 'real' safety profile of any medication (a) can be properly inferred only after the medication has been on the market long enough and has been used by large numbers of patients, and (b) is characterized by a continuous safety surveillance (see e.g. Yazici 2008).

This does not mean that some (negative) associated outcomes falls out of the scope of predictions and forecasts. But typically, an abundance of well-defined contrast classes is hard to come by. Cases of well-designed RCTs exist in which only a modest amount of possible future scenarios can be analytically and discretely discerned, predicted and forecast as plausible stories able to materialize in the future proceedings of the trial. What HR can do is ask for a broadening of the scope of scenarios in such a way that our imaginary and narrative practices take a larger role in attempts to discern and map out these alternatives. This is so not just because it would be hardly possible to detect such alternatives due to small effect sizes or their rarity, thus being left out of the radar of normalized probability distributions, but because of the inherent uncertainty involved in the trials themselves.

Uncertainty of future scenarios gathered from the standard protocols of RCTs is similar to well-known epistemological problems associated with Mill's methods for causality (Mill 1874). Similar to Mill's methods of causality, in fact, those protocols assume the *method of difference*. Assume that Jim enjoyed a dinner with his friends, eating the same food as the others, with the exception of the lobster plate. All his friends got ill but Jim did not. According to Mill's method, the lobster would be the factor more likely to be associated with the onset of the illness in question. Yet, it is evidently cumbersome to try to produce discrete scenarios from such situation and to determine that the lobster would, in general, be more likely associated with the illness for the other persons involved in the case. They could, for example, have developed resistance to the lobster's allergens. Of course, in this example there is no randomization, which is usually supposed to guarantee that both *known* and *unknown* confounding factors are distributed among the arms of the trial. Yet, this fact does not

---

[13] Typically, such RCTs are those in which it is unlikely that some unforeseen clinical conditions crop up, like for instance those aimed at corroboration of another large study that has already investigated the same clinical question. Even in these cases the effect sizes may vary, as the patient populations, cultures and clinical practices are far from being identical.

affect my argument, since randomization may also well fail to assess the reliability of causal judgments.[14]

In my view, what is problematic is to connect prospective alternate futures with all types of RCTs, since not *all* clinically relevant features, including all relevant endpoints, can be taken into consideration in the design of the trial. When conducting RCTs, there is plenty of room for unpredicted clinical situations and scenarios. Yet, even when the designer would welcome the use of alternate future scenarios, the uncertainty involved may be methodologically challenging or even paradoxical in case that new, unforeseen but relevant factors arise as future alternate scenarios are being narrated and imagined.

In the interpretation of CE as clinical agnosticism referred to in the previous section there is, besides the assumption of the alternate futures, a hidden assumption known as *the Principle of Indifference* (PoI) (Keynes 1921/63). This principle can be intuitively stated in the following way: given a number n of mutually exclusive and jointly exhaustive possibilities—none of which is favoured over the others by the available evidence –the probability of each possibility should be $1/n$. Given PoI, we come to assign the same probability to each alternative.

Assuming PoI means that clinical trials are subject to the statistical problem called *Bertrand's paradox*. A simple version of the paradox has been offered by van Fraassen (1989): imagine a factory that cuts iron cubes with constant edge-lengths ranging between 0 and 1 cm, and no other information is available. We want to know the probability that the next cube to be cut has edges between 0 and 0.5 cm in length. According to PoI, that probability is 1/2. Consider now the following question: what is the probability that the next cube will have a volume between 0 and 0.125 cm^3? If we apply PoI, then the answer is 1/8. But this is paradoxical in the sense that, based on the way evidence is presented, PoI comes to assign different probabilities to the same event class. In like manner, and as has recently been shown by Diamond and Geffen (2014), some innocent-sounding choices that assume PoI regarding the modes of randomization of a trial may in fact cause a biased allocation of patients. This—I want to emphasise—is due to the same reason as Bertrand's paradox. We are in an unequivocal predicament concerning the design of large studies. What is more, the implicit but illicit appeal to PoI also influences the choice of methods in reviews and meta-analyses.

The limitations of PoI were pointed out by Carnap (1955), who showed that the principle works only if we assume an ideal situation in which we can legitimately divide the reference class of individuals in a way that the only relevant properties among the groups of individuals are exactly the ones that we are considering: no other relevant features are allowed to contribute to how the groups of individuals are differentiated. But this is a condition virtually impossible to satisfy in actual clinical contexts (consider factors such as response to treatment, age groups, adjuvants used, co-morbidities, mortality, etc.; cf. Spector and Vesell 2006). In this light, we can say that the presence of residual uncertainty cannot be ruled out in clinical research. To

---

[14]For a discussion of another essential problem of RCTs, i.e. their external validity, see (Cartwright 2007).

put this into perspective, consider the following example made by Carnap (1966, pp. 24–25):

> Mr. Smith applies for life insurance. The company sends him to a doctor. The doctor reports that Smith has no serious diseases and that his birth certificate shows him to be forty years old. The company looks at its mortality tables; then, on the basis of the man's probable life expectancy, it offers him insurance at a certain rate. Mr. Smith may die before he reaches forty-one, or he may live to be a hundred. The probability of surviving one more year goes down and down as he gets older. Suppose he dies at forty-five. This is bad for the insurance company because he paid only a few premiums, and now they have to pay $20,000 to his beneficiary. Where are the equipossible cases? Mr. Smith may die at the age of forty, of forty –one, of forty-two, and so on. These are the possible cases. But they are not equipossible.

Carnap depicts here a case in which the possible outcomes cannot be classified as mutually exclusive and exhaustive cases fulfilling the condition of equipossibility. To bring this problem back to bear on the reliability of evidence from RCTs measured in terms of their statistical significance rates, the question is whether any such study alone shows any effect relevant to the justification of the principle of CE.

We can appreciate the impact of PoI in the context of a clinical decision case involving the choice from the set of mutually independent events. Smithson (2009) has presented an example which comes from the website of the Centre for Evidence-Based Medicine at the University of Toronto. A patient has been subjected to a serum ferritin test in order to help diagnose iron-deficiency anaemia. The test yields 40 mml/l. Let us consider two hypothetical scenarios depicted in Tables 10.1 and 10.2, respectively. In Table 10.1, a result equal or lower than 45 mml/l has the likelihood ratio of 8.24, and a post-test probability of 0.82 (70/85) of having the disease. Therefore, it seems rational to give the patient a proper treatment. In Table 10.2, with the same evidence base, the patient's test result has now the likelihood ratio of 0.76. This fact discourages to treat the patient. Thus, the way in which the

Table 10.1 First scenario

	Anaemia present	Anaemia absent	likelihood ratio
Result of the serum ferritin test			
(≤45 mmol/l)	70	15	8.24
(>45 mmol/l)	15	135	0.20
Total	85	150	

Table 10.2 Second scenario

	Anaemia present	Anaemia absent	likelihood ratio
Result of the serum ferritin test			
(≤35 mmol/l)	60	3	35.29
(>35 to ≤75 mmol/l)	15	35	0.76
(>75 mmol/l)	10	112	0.16
Total	85	150	

partition has been drawn up has a significant impact on the interpretation of one's clinical findings.

In conclusion, as soon as PoI is assumed, the justification of CE is clearly burdened by such methodological assumptions concerning the partitioning of the relevant event classes. To treat them as partitional is clearly a strong methodological assumption about the nature of uncertainty, which can have unexpected consequences. Fundamental uncertainty, in contrast, does not imply that the relevant search space could be neatly partitioned into event classes, as in such contexts we lack information about what the structure of the decision-making is in the first place.

This problem hampers also the new and otherwise promising methodology of hypothetical retrospection, as it relies on the notion of uncertainty that assumes the same principle. My analysis has pointed out that the assumption of UT involved in hypothetical retrospection, and similar other attempts to systematically connect uncertainty and moral permissibility such as CE, are meaningful only under the conditions in which (i) the future can be structured as a well-specified and finite range of alternate futures; (ii) all relevant factors associated with uncertainty for decision-making can be established; and (iii) no relevant factor may turn up along the way that would justify a different choice. It is however unlikely that all these three conditions be universally recognized and adhered to in the current and future practices of clinical research, or even that they reasonable could.[15]

10.4 Conclusion

The ethical justification of a trial is often assumed to be related to high epistemic standards that clinician-investigators hold concerning their ignorance, indifference and uncertainty on specific therapeutic choices. At the same time, ethical questions in medical research may benefit from being subject to critical scrutiny from epistemology and philosophy of science.

The criterion for the moral permissibility of ethical trials has traditionally been expressed under the framework of the principle of CE. The present chapter has proposed an analysis of different forms of CE. I showed that CE manifests principles

---

[15]There are some wider theoretical issues lurking at the back of these arguments, from which I here mention two: first, any uncritical or unrecognized presupposition of the PoI and the related confounding of risk-laden situations with fundamental uncertainty, is likely to have a negative impact on what the positive predictive values of large experimental studies are. This adds grist to Ionnadis's mill on replicability (Ionnadis 2005). Second, the practice of current clinical research is mainly frequentist. Would a Bayesian perspective on the design of RCTs be more suitable in handling (some variants of) CE, so as to turn it into an epistemic, quantifiable component obtained by prior elicitation of a Bayesian assessment of evidence? For instance, the notion of "admissibility of treatments" in a Bayesian trial may determine the restriction of possible treatments to a certain subgroup of subjects in order to ensure that a specific patient is not administered an inferior treatment (as judged by a committee of experts), merely for the reason that it would facilitate the completion of a trial (see Sedransk 1996). Yet, there are concerns on the epistemological and ethical validity and limits to such Bayesian approaches (see e.g. Teira 2010).

that rely on a hidden assumption of PoI. This is precisely why these principles fail as decision rules that can yield ethically uncompromised decisions across a variety of clinical contexts.

I then attempted to rehabilitate CE, beginning with the idea that uncertainty in future scenarios is characterized as a structure with well-specified alternative futures.[16] I showed that this attempt relies, in turn, on an unrestricted use of the PoI, and for that reason yields unwanted or even paradoxical conclusions. These conclusions undermine the level of prevailing epistemic standards and the trustworthiness of the processes by which the clinicians' beliefs and preferences come to be fixed.

What are the positive options? The development and application of the method of hypothetical retrospection, without the principle of UT that likewise relies on the PoI, may turn out to be promising. Some variants of CE might also be more convincing when embedded in alternative ethical theories and used as meta-principles in comparing different ethical theories. But even the supporters of CE must recognize that certain actions justified by CE are unethical, since they violate some other principles. Therefore, constraints to control the applicability of CE might need to be imposed. The values of such constraints may vary depending on the specific ethical theory one is prepared to embrace. CE might not be an infallible principle or a practical decision rule regulating uncertainty and moral leeway in a safe and sound way in every context; and yet, it may be—under specific conditions related to what I have called the constancy of alternate futures—a reasonable instrument for judging the levels of the moral permissibility of actions for different ethical theories under some specific and fixed levels of uncertainty. For instance, once the level of uncertainty remains invariant, ethical theories that are more tolerant than others may allow a greater set of permissible actions to be at the disposal of investigators. But be that as it may, such fixed levels of uncertainty are rarely present in everyday reality or in clinical research.

References

Annoni, M., Miller, F.G.: Placebos in clinical practice: an ethical overview. Douleur Anal. **27**(4), 215–220 (2014)

Bluhm, R.: The epistemology and ethics of chronic disease research: further lessons from ECMO. Theor Med Bioeth **31**(2), 107–122 (2010)

Broderick, J.P.: Devices and clinical trials. Overview and equipoise. Stroke **44**(Suppl 1), S3–S6 (2013)

Carnap, R.: Statistical and inductive probability. In: Statistical and Inductive Probability. Inductive Logic and Science. The Galois Institute of Mathematics and Art, Brooklyn (1955)

Carnap, R.: Introduction to the Philosophy of Science. Dover, New York (1966)

Cartwright, N.: Are RCTs the gold standard? BioSocieties **2**(1), 11–20 (2007)

Chiffi, D., Zanotti, R.: Fear of knowledge: clinical hypotheses in diagnostic and prognostic reasoning. J. Eval. Clin. Pract. **23**(5), 928–934 (2016)

---

[16]On the analysis of the role of uncertainty and future scenarios for clinical reasoning, see (Chiffi and Zanotti 2016).

Chiffi, D., Zanotti, R.: Knowledge and belief in placebo effect. J. Med. Philos. **42**(1), 70–85 (2017)

Chiffi, D., Pietarinen, A.V.: Fundamental uncertainty and values. Philosophia **45**(3), 1027–1037 (2017)

Diamond, A.D., Geffen, D.: Randomized trials, observational registries, and the foundations of evidence-based medicine. Am. J. Cardiol. **113**, 1436–1441 (2014)

Djulbegovic, B.: Articulating and responding to uncertainties in clinical research. J. Med. Philos. **32**(2), 79–98 (2007)

Emanuel, E.J., Wendler, D., Grady, C.: What makes clinical research ethical? JAMA **283**(20), 2701–2711 (2000)

Freedman, B.: Equipoise and the ethics of clinical research. N. Engl. J. Med. **317**(3), 141–145 (1987)

Freedman, B.: Value and validity as ethical requirements for research: a proposed explication. IRB: Eth. Hum. Res. **9**(6), 7–10 (1987b)

Fried, G.: Medical Experimentation: Personal Integrity and Social Policy. American Elsevier Publishing Co. Inc, , New York (1974)

Gigerenzer, G., Hoffrage, U., Kleinbolting, H.: Probabilistic mental models: a Brunswikian theory of confidence. Psychol. Rev. **98**, 506–528 (1991)

Gifford, F.: So-called "clinical equipoise" and the argument from design. J. Med. Philos. **32**(2), 135–150 (2007)

Hansson, S.O.: Hypothetical retrospection. . Eth. Theor. Moral Pract. **10**(2), 145–157 (2007)

Hansson, S.O.: From the casino to the jungle. Synthese **168**(3), 423–432 (2009)

Hansson, S.O.: The Ethics of Risk: Ethical Analysis in an Uncertain World. Palgrave Macmillan, New York (2013)

Howick, J.H.: The Philosophy of Evidence-Based Medicine. Wiley, London (2011)

Ioannidis, J.P.: Why most published research findings are false. PLoS Med. **2**(8), e124 (2005)

Karlawish, J.H.T., Lantos, J.: Community equipoise and the architecture of clinical research. Camb. Q. Healthc. Eths **6**, 385–396 (1997)

Keynes, J.M.: A Treatise on Probability. Macmillan, London (1921/1963)

Knight, F.H.: Risk, Uncertainty, and Profit. Hart, Schaffner & Marx; Houghton Mifflin Company, Boston (1921)

London, A.J.: Reasonable risks in clinical research: a critique and a proposal for the integrative approach. Stat. Med. **25**, 2869–2885 (2006)

London, A.J.: Clinical equipoise: foundational requirement or fundamental error? In: Steinbock, B. (ed.) The Oxford handbook of Bioethics, pp. 571–596. Oxford University Press, Oxford (2007)

Mill, J.S.: A System of Logic. Harper & Brothers, New York (1874)

Miller, F.G., Brody, H.: Clinical equipoise and the incoherence of research ethics. J. Med. Philos. **32**(2), 151–165 (2007)

Miller, F.G.: Equipoise and the dilemma of randomized clinical trials. N. Eng. J. Med. **346**(5), 476–480 (2011)

Miller, F.G.: Is anything lost if we give up clinical equipoise? Clin. Trials **9**, 632–633 (2012)

Miller, P.B., Weijer, C.: Rehabilitating equipoise. Kennedy Inst. Ethics J. **13**(2), 93–118 (2003)

Miller, P.B., Weijer, C.: Fiduciary obligation in clinical research. J. Law Med. Ethics **34**(2), 424–440 (2006)

Sackett, D.L.: Why randomized controlled trials fail but needn't: 1. Failure to gain "coal-face" commitment and to use the uncertainty principle. CMAJ **162**(9), 1311–1314 (2000)

Sedransk, N.: Admissibility of treatments. In: Kadane, J.B. (ed.) Bayesian Methods and Ethics in a Clinical Trial Design, pp. 65–113. Wiley, New York (1996)

Smithson, M.: How many alternatives? Partitions pose problems for predictions and diagnoses. Soc. Epistemol. **23**(3–4), 347–360 (2009)

Spector, R., Vesell, E.: Pharmacology and statistics: recommendations to strengthen a productive partnership. Pharmacology **78**, 113–122 (2006)

Stanev, R.: Early stopping of RCTs: two potential issues for error statistics. Synthese **192**, 1089–1116 (2015)

Teira, D.: Frequentist versus Bayesian clinical trials. In: Gifford, F. (ed.), Philosophy of Medicine, Volume 16. Handbook of the Philosophy of Science, pp. 255–297. Elsevier, Amsterdam (2010)

Tversky, A., Kahneman, D.: The framing of decisions and the psychology of choice. Science **211**, 453–458 (1981)

van Fraassen, B.: Laws and Symmetry. Oxford University Press, Oxford (1989)

Veach, R.M.: The irrelevance of equipoise. J. Med. Philos. **32**, 167–183 (2007)

Worrall, J.: Evidence and ethics in medicine. Perspect. Biol. Med. **51**(3), 418–431 (2008)

Yazici, Y.: Some concerns about adverse event reporting in randomized clinical trials. Bull. NYU Hosp. Jt. Dis. **66**(2), 143–145 (2008)

Chapter 11
Philosophical and Cognitive Elements of Risk Communication in Informed Consent

11.1 Introduction

Informed consent is a procedure by which a person agrees to undergo a medical treatment after discussing with doctors about the nature, indications, benefits and risks of that treatment (Davis et al. 2003). Through informed consent, moreover, the patient must also be informed about the risks and benefits associated with alternative treatments as well as about the risks and benefits of not undergoing the proposed treatment at all. This is especially important, since the number of therapeutic options now available for many diseases is increasing. On the one hand, we know that the patient needs to be treated with the best standard of care, while on the other, there is a need to validate new treatments which can be beneficial for present and future patients (Tobias and Souhami 1993). This situation may entail ethical problems in randomized clinical research that are related, as we have seen, to clinical equipoise. Consequently, it is of seminal importance for the doctor to explain to the patient all the main features of risk involved in the therapeutic options, and for the patient to understand the different scenarios caused by the various therapeutic options. In fact, the concepts of "risk" and "risk communication" turn out to be two key components of informed consent (Reynolds and Nelson 2007; Lloyd et al. 2001). Therefore, it seems necessary to connect the research on risk analysis and communication with the theme of informed consent. Furthermore, a philosophical and foundational standpoint may elucidate those aspects associated with risk communication that are usually neglected in the clinical practice of informed consent. The present problems connected with informed consent are not solely of a legal type, but also of an ethical nature. Although informed consent is intended to make sure, mainly from a legal point of view, that the patient fully understands the main features of the treatment and its consequences, it may fail in its practical application because of the problems connected to a patient's risk perception (Falagas et al. 2009; Lidz 2006; Fisher 2006).

D. Chiffi, *Clinical Reasoning: Knowledge, Uncertainty, and Values in Health Care*, Studies in Applied Philosophy, Epistemology and Rational Ethics 58, https://doi.org/10.1007/978-3-030-59094-9_11

Thus, a legally valid informed consent is by no means automatically ethically correct if the patient misunderstands the magnitude and the consequences of the risks and benefits of the treatment. From this perspective, a sound risk communication may clarify the ambiguities in a patient's health literacy.

The classical point of view in information theory is that communication must deal with a sender, a receiver and a channel of communication. Such model, though, does not fit with the demands of sound risk communication, since the doctor has to convey risk information by taking into account the way in which the patient may perceive it; and it is very likely that the patient will hold some initial prejudices concerning the intuitive evaluation of the risk. Thus, a different type of risk communication is required in which both doctor and patient try to promote a converging process of interpretation concerning the severity and the meaning of the risk. Such a converging process of interpretation needs to be free from cognitive and emotional biases: for this reason, it is necessary to be able to handle the main features that shape risk perception by means of "debiasing" techniques (Wills and Holmes-Rovner 2003).[1] From a philosophical point of view, this approach involves the construction of a framework in which communication is based on a meaning clarification and negotiation, which prove to be extremely relevant in health care. A similar framework can be found, for instance, in the theory of communication of the philosopher Donald Davidson (1986), who develops Paul Grice's ideas on dialogic conversation (Grice 1989) and assumes that communication succeeds if both speaker and hearer share passing theories of interpretation.

The acknowledgment of systematic errors due to biases and to the use of cognitive heuristics is also a very important tool for the constitution of converging strategies directed toward the interpretation of risk messages during the obtaining of informed consent. In addition, emotional and ethical themes related to health risk must be taken into consideration in this process, since they may deeply influence risk communication; in turn, risk communication shows to play a major role in the evaluation of the moral appropriateness of a therapy during the obtaining of informed consent (Doyal 2001, 2002). Thus, many features of a "subjective-person standard" (Holmes-Rovner and Wills 2002), which also deals with the biography and health literacy of a particular patient, may be added to some "debiasing" techniques in order to achieve an optimal level of risk communication during the informed consent procedure. Section 11.2 explores the definitions of risk, Sect. 11.3 investigates the main features of risk communication in health care, and Sect. 11.4 analyses the role of social and individual factors in risk perception. Then, Sect. 11.5 deals with the framing of probabilistic information for health risks, whereas the many facets of the qualitative presentation of risk are pointed out in Sect. 11.6. Section 11.7 deals with ethical and affective features of risk communication, and finally Sect. 11.8 concludes the chapter.

---

[1]It is worth noting that not all types of bias can be considered as errors in reasoning. Quite often, cognitive biases have an evolutionistic justification which may be useful for heuristic forms of (economic, abductive and practical) reasoning (Woods 2012).

11.2 Defining Risk

Even though there is no unique and universally accepted notion of "risk" (Aven and Renn 2009; Hampel 2006; Hansson 2010), a classical definition, as we have seen, describes it as the probability of an (uncertain) outcome, which might occur (or not) during a specific time period, in combination with the magnitude of the effect and its consequences (Royal Society 1982). Such a definition of risk can embrace different scenarios, i.e. a low-probability risk having severe consequences with a high-probability risk bringing about modest consequences in the same lapse of time.[2] Yet, it is worth quoting Rosa: "despite the still rapidly growing literature on the topic of risk there is remarkably little consensus over what, in fact, is meant by risk" (Rosa 2001).

The debate ranges from positions where risk is considered as a state of the world, independent of percipient actors, which is an objective point of view (Cohen 2003), to others which assume that risk corresponds to its perception, viz. risk conceived from a mere subjective point of view (Jasanoff 1999). Neither of these two opposite conceptions fully encompasses the complexity of risk. On the one hand, a risk cannot be completely independent of the perceiving subject, since an outcome that does not have any impact on humans cannot be conceived as a risk, but rather as a hazard or a potential harm. Only when an individual is exposed to a hazard can a risk be determined based on the severity of the same. Moreover, the vulnerability of the individual to the risk of a single exposure should not be confused with the cumulative risk of many exposures. On the other hand, a risk cannot merely be present in people's minds without any external counterpart. Risk indeed is a multidimensional notion which is explained both by subjective and objective factors: e.g. if there is an explosion in a location X, then we know that a hazard exists, but there is no risk if no individual is near X or if the explosion does not cause any indirect harm for individuals. Furthermore, both facts and values jointly play a part in the determination of risk, since both normative and descriptive features explain its complexity (Hansson 2010). In particular, the systematic deviation of descriptive 'models' from the normative ones—due to cognitive and emotional biases and social factors—shows the inextricability of the concept of risk.

11.3 Defining Risk Communication

The definition of risk communication is also problematic. As observed by Ruhrmann, "risk communication can be defined as a process that increases the selectivity of the perception and communication of decision consequences" (Ruhrmann 2008,

---

[2]In the field of disaster risk assessment, the following are identified as risk components: the potential danger (hazard), the exposed value (or exposure), and the vulnerability, which can be defined as the susceptibility of the exposed elements (people, manufactured products, economic activities, etc.) to suffer damage caused by a specific potentially harmful event (UNISDR 2015).

p. 4415). In order to gain more insight and better understand how to tackle with the hardships of risk communication, there are multiple models that can be used. It is acknowledged in the health domain that "good communication with patients can be associated with improved treatment adherence and physician communication styles appear to be associated with the risk of malpractice litigation" (Ihler 2003). Communicating with patients and involving them in decision-making is also considered a doctor's duty from a deontological standpoint (Godolphin 2003): in fact, the paternalistic view according to which doctors should assume a dominant position over patients for any decision is no longer plausible and permissible. Thus, risk communication in the doctor-patient interaction must be embedded in a relationship-based and person-centred model, in which the doctor expresses a clinical point of view and any possible biases are pondered through dialogue with the patient (Rubinelli and Schulz 2006). But in many concrete contexts, this dialogic strategy cannot be followed, e.g. when there is an emergency intervention or when there exists only one medical care strategy. Moreover, not all patients might appreciate the democratic dialogic approach, preferring a one-way communication (Collins and Street 2009), which is also why a universally valid model of risk communication does not exist. Nonetheless, "the fact that patients may say that they want their clinicians to make final decisions about their care does not mean that they do not want to be involved in it" (Doyal 2002, p. 104).

A doctor, then, must be capable of imagining a patient's risk perception by researching all of the possible biases that can cause a breakdown of communication or a wrong interpretation of the risk magnitude. A doctor's ability to avoid cognitive and emotional biases will influence the patient's risk perception and prevent the occurrence of additional risk due to ineffective risk communication (Gray and Ropeik 2002).

11.4 Risk Perception

We will now consider the most frequent biases and factors affecting risk perception, with the knowledge that the scientific and normative explication of risk is partially inadequate for understanding the way in which risk is assessed by lay people. Indeed, many factors contribute to modify the individual and social 'perception of risk'. The discrepancies found between normative and descriptive models of risk assessment are due to risk perception being associated with risk acceptance, which is in turn strongly affected by the psychology of risk perception and evaluation (Starr and Whipple 1980). This issue is fundamental for informed consent, since if the doctor can (at least partially) foresee how the medical information will be elaborated by the patient, the doctor-patient communication will be more person-centred, and therefore more effective.

Recently, it has been acknowledged that two cognitive processes influence decision-making, namely System 1, which is fast, automatic, and difficult to control, and System 2, which is slower, serial and very controlled. System 2 is necessary to control the cognitive and emotional heuristics and biases of System 1 associated with risk perception (Kahneman 2003). Hence, both systems are involved in the information processing of risk perception. Let us consider the main biases and factors affecting risk perception which are essential features of System 1.

The first contemporary paper on risk perception (written in 1969) dealt with the technological risk of nuclear power (Starr 1969), but more recent literature on the issue is very rich (for a comprehensive review see (Renn 2008a, b)). For sound and successful risk communication it is of paramount importance to acknowledge those factors that entail a significant distance between a scientific and objective explication of risk and its public perception (Slovic 1987; Fischhoff et al., 1978; Breakwell 2000). People are likely to undervalue the risk of common harms (e.g. cancer and diabetes) and to overrate risks with low probability or with severe consequences (the so-called "compression error in risk estimation") (Alaszewski and Horlick-Jones 2003).

Factors related to the nature of the risk in risk perception are the following: "new risk", "dreaded risk", "number of exposures" and "unnatural and immoral risk" (Sjöberg 2000a). At any rate, it is also necessary to understand whether the perceived risk has a general or personal target, since there is a considerable difference between these two kinds of risk. The four factors contributing to risk perception explain 60/70% of its variance for a general risk, whilst they explain only 20% of individual risk. In addition, the secondary factors affecting risk perception such as trust in the risk communicators (e.g. experts, institutions, governments, etc.) count for 9% of the variance in the perception of risk; and cultural factors contribute to 5% of the variance. What follows from these findings is that the assessment of individual risk is one of the challenging questions of risk perception, since there is a great reduction in the association between the aforementioned four factors and personal risk. For instance, individualised risk estimation of breast cancer by means of the Gail model shows many methodological limitations, since it is not easy to switch from probabilities expressing risk factors about a general outcome to an individualised probability of a personal outcome (Holmberg and Parascandola 2010). Then, when evaluating personal risk related to common activities, people are more likely to be influenced by an optimistic bias (also known as unrealistic optimism) (Weinstein 1989), due to a distortion in the perception of personal vulnerability with respect to a hazard. By way of example, let us consider the following scenario. Even though the connection between sun exposition and skin cancer is widely known by the public, people are not able to estimate their vulnerability: they generally underestimate the incidence of skin cancer cases due to sun-related behaviours, since common risks are considered preventable and controllable, especially when they are voluntary (Branstrom et al. 2006). By contrast, a pessimistic bias is usually acknowledged in people with depressive symptoms (Strunk et al. 2006; Moore and Fresco 2007). This just goes to show how difficult judging and evaluating personal risk is.

11.5   Framing Information About Risk

The way in which doctor-patient communication is framed may have an effect on the shift from risk aversion to risk taking and vice versa, due to some heuristics (such as framing effect, anchoring and availability heuristics), which can result in cognitive biases modifying the rationality of probabilistic decision-making (Tversky and Kahneman 1974, 1981; Klein 2005). The framing of the outcomes in risky decisions can change the perception of risk because people usually prefer decisions presented under a positive rather than a negative frame, or also because patients may not understand during informed consent why the choice of a treatment x is better than a treatment y. By way of example, a survival rate of 80% may be conceived as less risky than a death rate of 20%. People are more likely to maximize gains when the information is presented in a positive framework (e.g. lives saved), and to minimize losses when they are framed in a negative context (e.g. lives lost) (Kahneman and Tversky 1979). In the health domain, it has been observed that the message describing the benefits related to illness prevention such as condom use and sunscreen are more effective when framed in a positive way, while a message related to a procedure for detecting an illness such as mammography is more effective when the message describes the negative aspects of non-adherence to therapy. Detection behaviours, in fact, are perceived as particularly risky because they might negatively change the life of the individual in the short run, even if in the long run the objective risk can be reduced; prevention behaviours, instead, usually involve a future hazard which is not perceived as very risky at the moment (Rothman and Salovey 1997). This suggests that the choice of time interval is a key component of risk perception: a present harm is considered more threatening than a harm of the same severity in the future (Bogardus et al. 1999).

In addition, there may be an overestimation of an outcome's risk when its assessment is based on another related event that is familiar to the decision maker (*anchoring heuristic*): for example, physicians might be less likely to prescribe warfarin to patients with atrial fibrillation after one case of a severe adverse bleeding event caused by warfarin has taken place (Choudhry et al. 2006). Furthermore, the formal property of the message may also change the perception of the risk itself and, consequently, the effectiveness of risk communication. For instance, if a therapy reduces the probability of an adverse outcome from 20 to 15%, then the absolute risk reduction is 5% while the relative risk reduction is 25%. In such situations, it may happen that patients would more likely decide to undergo the therapy when the risk reduction is presented in the relative form rather than in the absolute mode (Gordon-Lubitz 2003). The issue of presenting such risk evaluations in relative terms is also evident when dealing with the concept of "relative risk" (RR). RR provides the ratio of the probability (incidence in epidemiological terms) of the disease in the exposed population (IE) to that in the unexposed population (IU), while the absolute risk reduction (ARR) is the measure of association based on the absolute difference between IE and IU. By way of example, consider the case where IU is very small, say equal to 0.0001 and RR = 3: still ARR may be insignificant, being equal to 0.0002

(Jardine and Hrudey 1997). Communicating only RR can be misleading, since people neglect base rates. Consequently, in some contexts it can be useful—and it is indeed recommended—to present data in accordance with the concept of "number needed to treat (NNT)" rather than by means of probabilities. NNT is defined as 1/ARR and expresses the number of patients who need to be treated in order to avoid one additional outcome. In the previous example, NNT is in fact 5000.

Yet, when risks are presented as relative frequencies using larger numbers rather than percentages, they are perceived as even more dangerous. A mortality of 1286 out of 10,000 has been reported to be perceived as more hazardous than 24%, but this is paradoxical since a percentage of 12.86% is perceived as more dangerous than a percentage of 24% (Yamagishi 1997). In any case, a wrong interpretation of probabilistic data and tests is very frequent, even among physicians, since they may confuse the *sensitivity* of a test (i.e. the proportion of people with the disease who correctly present a true positive result for the test) with the *positive predictive value* (i.e. the proportion of individuals with positive test results who are correctly diagnosed) (Hoffrage et al. 2000; Eddy 1982). It is also very common for physicians (as well as for other people) not to take into consideration the a priori probabilities in the assessment of the probability of an outcome. Likewise, the probability of a conjunction may be estimated exceeding the probability of its constituents (conjunction fallacy), thus violating the axioms of probability calculus (Tversky and Kahneman 1983).

The assessment of the probability of a decision also depends on the order in which the alternatives are presented: when physicians or policy decision-makers must choose between two different medical options A and B, they assign two probabilities to the outcomes of A and B. When adding a new alternative, C, quite similar (but not identical) to A or B, they can increase the probability assigned to A or B or can maintain the initial assessments of probabilities of A and B, which seems paradoxical.[3] Therefore, the order and the frame by which the alternatives are presented in decision-making has a non-marginal impact on the assessment of the probabilities associated with different outcomes (Redelmeier and Shafir 1995). An analogous phenomenon is the *comparative ignorance hypothesis* (Fox and Tversky 1995), which states that ambiguity aversion (Ellsberg 1961; Wakker 2000), occurring in decision contexts in which people are more likely to gamble on *known* rather than unknown probabilities,[4] is present if people assess the known and the unknown prospects jointly; otherwise such ambiguity aversion is not very evident anymore.

---

[3]Of course, we are assuming that the probability of C is different from zero. Remember that in the probability calculus the possibility space Ω of all alternatives must sum up to 1.

[4]When probabilities are unknown, we are in the contest of fundamental uncertainty (Chiffi and Pietarinen 2017).

11.6   Qualitative Presentation of Risk

Risk is often not merely an issue concerning the cognitive assessment of probability; as a consequence, heuristics are sometimes hard to apply to concrete cases of risk perception (Sjöberg 2000a). This happens also because social factors may provide an amplification or attenuation of public risk assessment (Kasperson et al. 1988). In fact, risk perception does not occur in a social vacuum (Breakwell 2000): in many cases the public perception of risk has to deal with social stigma (namely when the perception of a risk is associated with events that are very dreaded or with unknown consequences), and the phenomenon or activity receives wide and negative coverage by the media. For example, the public perception of blood transfusion is still affected by the stigma connected with the risk of contracting HIV/AIDS (Finucane et al. 2000a, b). Media information can thus increase the level of stigma, only to become a new factor for public risk perception. Yet, the attribution of a level of social trust to different kinds of communication can reduce such stigma: medical sources, for instance, can play a relevant role in this context, as they are commonly more trusted than the governmental and institutional ones (Frewer and Miles 2003).

Mass media generally present messages about risk in a qualitative way. Such a qualitative presentation of the probability associated with a risk is very problematic, since people tend to overestimate the probabilities associated with expressions like "common risk" and "rare risk" (Knapp et al. 2004). The understanding of a message such as "there is some possibility of success" is not equivalent to the understanding provided when saying "it is quite uncertain that it will succeed" (Hilton 2008). Furthermore, it is more convenient to use graphical displays of information about risk rather than probabilistic data, since graphs increase the effectiveness of risk perception and communication (Edwards et al. 2002). Especially in the context of informed consent, people do not even understand the design of the study. The words "randomized clinical trials", "double-blinding" and "random assignment" may sound meaningless if they are not analytically explained. Consequently, enrolling patients in a study whose design is not understood by them may imply some ethical problems which connect scientific research with medical ethics.

11.7   Informed Consent and Risk Communication:
Emotional and Ethical Themes

Despite the assumption that morality is partially missing from much of the work on risk perception (Sjöberg 2000b), it is undeniable that the quality dimension of risk perception is often associated with ethical and emotional factors. Mass health communication campaigns and the choice of how to frame information are issues connected with emotional and ethical themes: these external aspects are in fact able to shape risk perception and, consequently, to influence the final decision of undergoing a treatment or not. Notably, emotion, in the form of affect, plays a substantial role in risk perception and communication (Slovic et al. 2004, 2005). Affect is a polar concept experienced as a feeling state sensitive to positive or negative quality of stimuli, i.e. related to goodness or badness, happiness or sadness. Quite surprisingly, affect in the perception of risk seems to show some similarities with the notion of 'thin moral concept' in meta-ethics (Williams 1972). Examples of thin moral concepts are: bad or good, right or wrong; while more complex moral concepts which do not show a polar structure are named 'thick moral concepts': courageous, cruel, etc.[5]

Affect seems to explain the inverse relationship between perceived risk and perceived benefit, since if an activity like vaccination is associated with a positive affect, then the risk related to vaccination is practically neglected; on the other side, if something is connected to a negative affect such as nuclear power, then the risks are taken into account while the benefits may be easily neglected. More in general, if an activity is presented by describing its increasing level of benefit (or risk), then the level of perceived risk (or benefit) decreases; conversely, if an activity is presented by describing its decreasing level of benefit (or risk), then the level of perceived risk (or benefit) increases (Finucane et al. 2000a, b). In other words, it seems that people make decisions not just about what they think but also about what they feel (Slovic et al. 2002). This is a seminal aspect for risk communication, since the information associated with the risks or the benefits of an activity is determined by the particular type of perceived affect (Greene and Haidt 2002; Loewenstein 2001). This distinction between cognitive and emotional judgments may resemble the distinction between hedonistic theories and preference-based theories in ethics, but further research is needed to clarify this issue.

Socio-demographic factors also influence the estimated severity of the impact of affect. For instance, in health, recreational and gambling domains, women show a lower tendency of engaging in risky activities, whereas there is no significant difference with regard to social risks (Harris et al. 2006). Moreover, the assessment of risk and the understanding of risk communication in older adults are both deeply influenced by affect, compared with younger people (Finucane 2008). Thus, the ethical and emotional dimension of risk perception and communication, mediated by socio-demographic factors, plays a primary role in risk taking and risk aversion. Neglecting the patient's risk perception, emotions and biography (socioeconomic status, educational level, etc.) may well lead to a breakdown of communication between the doctor and the patient in the decision-making concerning the treatment options during the informed consent process, thus undermining the person-centred approach.

---

[5]On the relation between risk, values and normative constraints, see (Chiffi and Giaretta 2014). For a pragmatist view on risk and values in science, see (Chiffi and Pietarinen 2019).

11.8   Conclusion

The communication of health-related risk is particularly complex, because of the multiplicity of factors shaping risk perception and communication. Moreover, decisions made under conditions of uncertainty are influenced by many biases and, consequently, "feel wrong psychologically" (Round 2001; Balla et al. 1989). Thus, risk (and decision) analysis seems to be an elusive issue. Recently, ethical and emotional features of risk have been gradually integrated with the cognitive (psychometric) program in risk perception. These new trends in risk perception and communication are very important for the debate on informed consent, since the latter needs to be not only legally, but also morally valid, and requires good clinical practice. This purpose can also be achieved by means of sound risk communication. In fact, we have observed that poor communication of risks can lead to the adoption of potentially dangerous treatment options, imposing harm without the patient's informed consent; this is morally unacceptable and violates patient autonomy. Providing complete information to the patient is a necessary but insufficient condition for a substantial understanding of the therapeutic options that may be presented in the informed consent process.[6] First, it is necessary to use 'debiasing' techniques in order to prevent cognitive and emotional biases or, alternatively, to be able to take advantages from their consideration in clinical reasoning. Secondly, when communicating with the patient, the doctor needs to keep in mind that the informed consent is directed towards an individual person who has a unique biography, personal prejudices and world view. Doctors, nurses and patients may achieve converging interpretation strategies concerning the most satisfactory therapeutic option after having chosen the right frame to present the risks and the benefits of the treatments. Thus, it is of paramount importance that the ethics of risk communication be associated with appropriate communicative strategies which trace their origins in the philosophy of risk. Philosophy, indeed, can very well contribute to the epistemological and ethical aspects of clinical practice in the understanding and communication of risk. As such, it is central to the development of the much-valued person-centred and humanistic paradigm in health care.

References

Alaszewski, A., Horlick-Jones, T.: How can doctors communicate information about risk more effectively? BMJ **327**(7417), 728–731 (2003)

Aven, T., Renn, O.: On risk defined as an event where the outcome is uncertain. J. Risk Res. **12**(1), 1–11 (2009)

Balla, J.I., Elstein, A.S., Christensen, C.: Obstacles to acceptance of clinical decision analysis. BMJ **298**(6673), 579–582 (1989)

---

[6]This is particularly true for innovative fields in biomedicine regarding, for instance, research biobanks (Sanchini et al. 2016) in which risks are better exemplified by fundamental uncertainties permeating future health technologies.

Bogardus, S.T., Holmboe, E., Jr., Jekel, J.F.: Perils, pitfalls, and possibilities in talking about medical risk. J. Am. Med. Assoc. **281**(11), 1037–1041 (1999)

Branstrom, R., Kristjansson, S., Ullen, H.: Risk perception, optimistic bias, and readiness to change sun related behaviour. Eur. J. Pub. Health **16**(5), 492–497 (2006)

Breakwell, G.M.: Risk communication: factors affecting impact. Br. Med. Bull. **56**(1), 110–120 (2000)

Chiffi, D., Giaretta, P.: Normative facets of risk. Epistemologia **37**(2), 217–233 (2014)

Chiffi, D., Pietarinen, A.V.: Fundamental uncertainty and values. Philosophia **45**(3), 1027–1037 (2017)

Chiffi, D., Pietarinen, A.V.: Risk and values in science: a Peircean view. Axiomathes **29**(4), 329 346 (2019)

Choudhry, N.K., Anderson, G.M., Laupacis, A., Ross- Degnan, D., Normand, S.T., Soumerai, S.B.: Impact of adverse events on prescribing warfarin in patients with atrial fibrillation: matched pair analysis. BMJ **332**(7534), 141–145 (2006)

Cohen, B.L.: Probabilistic risk analysis for a high-level radioactive waste repository. Risk Anal. **23**(5), 909–915 (2003)

Collins, D.L., Street, R.L., Jr.: A dialogic model of conversations about risk: Coordinating perceptions and achieving quality decisions in cancer care. Soc. Sci. Med. **68**(8), 1506–1512 (2009)

Davidson, D.: A nice derangement of epitaphs. In: LePore, E. (ed.) Truth and Interpretation: Perspectives on the Philosophy of Donald Davidson, pp. 433–446. Basil Blackwell, Oxford (1986)

Davis, N., Pohlman, A., Gehlbach, B., Kress, J.P., McAtee, J., Herlitz, J., Hall, J.: Improving the process of informed consent in the critically Ill. J. Am. Med. Assoc. **289**(15), 1963–1968 (2003)

Doyal, L.: Informed consent: moral necessity or illusion? Qual. in Health Care **10**(Supplement 1), i29–i33 (2001)

Doyal, L.: Good clinical practice and informed consent are inseparable. Heart **87**(2), 103–105 (2002)

Eddy, D.M.: Probabilistic reasoning in clinical medicine: problems and opportunities. In: Kahneman, D., Slovic, P., Tversky, A. (eds.) Judgment Under Uncertainty: Heuristics and Bias, pp. 249–267. Cambridge University Press, Cambridge (1982)

Edwards, A., Elwyn, G., Mulley, A.: Explaining risks: turning numerical data into meaningful pictures. BMJ **324**(7341), 827–830 (2002)

Ellsberg, D.: Risk, ambiguity, and the savage axioms. Quart. J. Econ. **75**(4), 643–669 (1961)

Falagas, M.E., Korbila, I.P., Giannopoulou, K.P., Kindilis, B.K., Peppas, G.: Informed consent: how much and what do patients understand? Am. J. Surg. **198**(3), 420–435 (2009)

Finucane, M.L.: Emotion, affect, and risk communication with older adults: challenges and opportunities. J. Risk Res. **11**(8), 983–997 (2008)

Finucane, M.L., Alhakami, A., Slovic, P., Johnson, S.M.: The affect heuristic in judgments of risks and benefits. J. Behav. Decis. Mak. **13**(1), 1–17 (2000a)

Finucane, M.L., Slovic, P., Mertz, C.K.: Public perception of the risk of blood transfusion. Transfusion **40**(8), 1017–1022 (2000b)

Fischhoff, B., Slovic, P., Lichtenstein, S., Read, S., Combs, B.: How safe is safe enough? A psychometric study of attitudes towards technological risks and benefits. Policy Sci. **9**(2), 127–152 (1978)

Fisher, J.A.: Procedural misconceptions and informed consent: Insights from empirical research on the clinical trials Industry. Kennedy Inst. Ethics J. **16**(3), 251–268 (2006)

Fox, C.R., Tversky, A.: Ambiguity Aversion and Comparative Ignorance. Quart. J. Econ. **110**(3), 585–603 (1995)

Frewer, L.J., Miles, S.: Temporal stability of the psychological determinants of trust: Implications for communication about food risks. Health Risk Soc. **5**(3), 259–271 (2003)

Godolphin, W.: The role of risk communication in shared decision making. BMJ **327**(7417), 692–693 (2003)

Gordon-Lubitz, R.J.: Risk communication: problems of presentation and understanding. J. Am. Med. Assoc. **28**(1), 95 (2003)

Gray, G.M., Ropeik, D.P.: Dealing with the dangers of fear: the role of risk communication. Health Aff. **21**(6), 106–116 (2002)

Greene, J., Haidt, J.: How (and where) does moral judgment work? Trends Cognit. Sci. **6**(12), 517–523 (2002)

Grice, H.P.: Studies in the Way of Words. Harvard University Press, Cambridge, Mass (1989)

Hampel, J.: Different concepts of risk—A challenge for risk communication. Int. J. Med. Microbiol. **296**(Supplement 40), 5–10 (2006)

Hansson, S.O.: Risk: objective or subjective, facts or values. J. Risk Res. **13**(2), 231–238 (2010)

Harris, C.R., Jenkins, M., Glaser, D.: Gender differences in risk assessment: why do women take fewer risks than men? Judgment Decis. Mak. J. **1**(1), 48–63 (2006)

Hilton, D.: Emotional tone and argumentation in risk communication. Judgment Decis. Mak. J. **3**(1), 100–110 (2008)

Hoffrage, U., Lindsey, S., Hertwig, R., Gigerenzer, G.: MEDICINE: communicating statistical information. Science **290**(5500), 2261–2262 (2000)

Holmberg, C., Parascandola, M.: Individualised risk estimation and the nature of prevention. Health Risk Soc. **12**(5), 441–452 (2010)

Holmes-Rovner, M., Wills, C.E.: Improving informed consent: insights from behavioral decision research. Med. Care **4**(9), V-30–V-38

Ihler, E.: Patient-physician communication. J. Am. Med. Assoc. **289**(1), 92 (2003)

Jardine, C.G., Hrudey, S.E.: Mixed messages in risk communication. Risk Anal. **17**(4), 489–498 (1997)

Jasanoff, S.: The songlines of risk. Environ. Values **8**(2), 135–152 (1999)

Kahneman, D., Tversky, A.: Prospect theory: an analysis of decision under risk. Econometrica **47**(2), 263–291 (1979)

Kahneman, D.: Maps of bounded rationality: a perspective on intuitive judgment and choice. In: Frängsmyr, T. (ed.) Les Prix Nobel: The Nobel Prizes 2002, pp. 449–489. Nobel Foundation, Stockholm (2003)

Kasperson, R.E., Renn, O., Slovic, P., Brown, H.S., Emel, J., Goble, R., Kasperson, J.X., Ratick, S.: The social amplification of risk a conceptual framework. Risk Anal. **8**(2), 177–187 (1988)

Klein, J.G.: Five pitfalls in decisions about diagnosis and prescribing. BMJ **330**(7494), 781–783 (2005)

Knapp, P., Raynor, D.K., Berry, D.C.: Comparison of two methods of presenting risk information to patients about the side effects of medicines. Qual. Safety Health Care **13**(3), 176–180 (2004)

Lidz, C.W.: The therapeutic misconception and our models of competency and informed consent. Behav. Sci. Law **24**(4), 535–546 (2006)

Lloyd, A., Hayes, P., Bell, P.R.F., Naylor, A.R.: The role of risk and benefit perception in informed consent for surgery. Med. Decis. Mak. **21**(2), 141–149 (2001)

Loewenstein, G.F., Weber, E.U., Hsee, C.K., Welch, N.: Risk as feelings. Psychol. Bull. **127**(2), 267–286 (2001)

Moore, M.T., Fresco, D.M.: Depressive realism and attributional style: implications for individuals at risk for depression. Behav. Ther. **38**(2), 144–154 (2007)

Redelmeier, D.A., Shafir, E.: Medical decision-making in situations that offer multiple alternatives. J. Am. Med. Assoc. **273**(4), 302–305 (1995)

Renn, O.: Concepts of risk: an interdisciplinary review - Part 1: Disciplinary risk concepts. Gaia-Ecol. Perspect. Sci. Soc. **17**(1), 50–66 (2008a)

Renn, O.: Concepts of risk: An interdisciplinary review—Part 2: integrative approaches. Gaia-Ecol. Perspect. Sci. Soc. **17**(2), 196–204 (2008b)

Reynolds, W.W., Nelson, R.M.: Risk perception and decision processes underlying informed consent to research participation. Soc. Sci. Med. **65**(10), 2105–2115 (2007)

Rosa, E.A.: Metatheoretical foundations for post-normal risk. J. Risk Res. **1**(1), 15–44 (2001)

Rothman, A.J., Salovey, P.: Shaping perceptions to motivate healthy behavior: the role of message framing. Psychol. Bull. **121**(1), 3–19 (1997)

Round, A.: Introduction to clinical reasoning. J. Eval. Cli. Pract. **7**(2), 109–117 (2001)

Royal-Society: Risk: Analysis, Perception, and Management. Report of a Royal Society Study Group. Royal Society, London (1982)

Rubinelli, S., Schulz, P.J.: "Let Me Tell You Why!". When argumentation in doctor-patient interaction makes a difference. Argumentation **20**(3), 353–375 (2006)

Ruhrmann, G.: Risk Communication. In: Donsbach, W. (ed.) International Encyclopedia of Communication, pp. 4415–4419. Wiley, Oxford (2008)

Sanchini, V., Bonizzi, G., Disalvatore, D., Monturano, M., Pece, S., Viale, G., Di Fiore, P.P., Boniolo, G.: A trust-based pact in research biobanks. From theory to practice. Bioethics **30**(4), 260–271 (2016)

Sjöberg, L.: Factors in risk perception. Risk Anal. **20**(1), 1–11 (2000a)

Sjöberg, L.: The methodology of risk perception research. Qual. Quant. **34**(4), 407–418 (2000b)

Slovic, P.: Perception of risk. Science **236**(4799), 280–285 (1987)

Slovic, P., Finucane, M., Peters, E., MacGregor, D.G.: Rational actors or rational fools: implications of the affect heuristic for behavioral economics. J. Soc.-Econ. **31**(4), 329–342 (2002)

Slovic, P., Finucane, M.L., Peters, E., MacGregor, D.G.: Risk as analysis and risk as feelings: some thoughts about affect, reason, risk, and rationality. Risk Anal. **24**(2), 311–322 (2004)

Slovic, P., Peters, E., Finucane, M.L., MacGregor, D.G.: Affect, risk, and decision making. Health Psychol. **24**(Supplement 4), S35–S40 (2005)

Starr, C.: Social benefit versus technological risk. Science **165**(899), 1232–1238 (1969)

Starr, C., Whipple, C.: Risks of risk decisions. Science **208**(4448), 1114–1119 (1980)

Strunk, D.R., Lopez, H., De Rubeis, R.J.: Depressive symptoms are associated with unrealistic negative predictions of future life events. Behav. Res. Ther. **44**(6), 861–882 (2006)

Tobias, J.S., Souhami, R.L.: Fully informed consent can be needlessly cruel. BMJ **307**(6913), 1199–1201 (1993)

Tversky, A., Kahneman, D.: Judgment under Uncertainty: heuristics and Biases. Science **185**(4157), 1124–1131 (1974)

Tversky, A., Kahneman, D.: The framing of decisions and the psychology of choice. Science **211**(4481), 453–458 (1981)

Tversky, A., Kahneman, D.: Extensional versus intuitive reasoning: the conjunction fallacy in probability judgment. Psychol. Rev. **90**(4), 293–315 (1983)

United Nations Office for Disaster Risk Reduction (UNISDR): UNISDR Annual Report 2015: 2014–15 Biennium Work Programme Final Report, Geneva. https://www.unisdr.org/files/48588_unisdrannualreport2015evs.pdf (2015)

Wakker, P.P.: Uncertainty aversion: a discussion of critical issues in health economics. Health Econ. **9**(3), 261–263 (2000)

Weinstein, N.D.: Optimistic biases about personal risks. Science **246**(4935), 1232–1233 (1989)

Williams, B.A.O: Morality: An Introduction to Ethics. Harper & Row, New York (1972)

Wills, C.E., Holmes-Rovner, M.: Patient comprehension of information for shared treatment decision making: state of the art and future directions. Patient Educ. Couns. **50**(3), 285–290 (2003)

Woods, J.: Cognitive economics and the logic of abduction. Rev. Symbolic Logic **5**(1), 148–161 (2012)

Yamagishi, K.: When a 12.86% mortality is more dangerous than 24.14%: implications for risk communication. Appl. Cognit. Psychol **11**(6), 495–506 (1997)

Chapter 12
Concluding Thoughts: Towards a Clinical Philosophy

With this book I tried to emphasise that philosophy may greatly contribute to sound clinical reasoning. The philosophy of health care usually focuses on bioethics and philosophy of medicine, but fails to pay attention to the valuable contributions that clinicians outside the medical world can give. The reason behind this tendency may still rely on the strength of the classical biomedical model of care, in which the idiographic nature of care is not always fully investigated. As a way of example, I showed that the placebo effect can hardly be explained within a biomedical model, which is exclusively based on the pathophysiological conditions of care; instead, such peculiar phenomenon may be better defined within the confines of the nursing practice. In this light, the first part of the book provides a critical evaluation of the structure and logical nature of diagnostic and prognostic judgments in health care, whereas the second part presents an analysis of the nature of clinical knowledge from a nursing perspective, which underlies the critical elements of many classical nursing theories.

Upon the formulation of a clinical judgment, a common clinical issue to stumble upon usually consists in trying to find a meaningful reference class in population studies and to 'particularize' the relevant clinical factors of that class to a specific patient (Fuller and Flores 2015). This clinical attitude may be problematic. First, as the epidemiological evidence may be difficult to amalgamate and replicate in different sources, it is not rare to have to deal with a great amount of uncertainty.[1] Second, isolating the reference class for a patient in a population, as we have seen, may be extremely challenging given the high number of relevant factors involved when making a clinical judgment. And finally, the patient's preferences and values

---

[1] It is quite common to have great heterogeneity among different studies evaluated in meta-analysis. A recent proposal to adjust the measure of heterogeneity in virtue of the statistical power of individual studies is (Berchialla et al. 2020).

D. Chiffi, *Clinical Reasoning: Knowledge, Uncertainty, and Values in Health Care*, Studies in Applied Philosophy, Epistemology and Rational Ethics 58, https://doi.org/10.1007/978-3-030-59094-9_12

may contribute to shaping clinical judgment. This is a common way of reasoning when making a diagnosis, a prognosis and selecting the options of care. For several reasons, this process can hardly be mechanized in all regards. In fact, even though taxonomical tools and protocols used for diagnosis or prognosis may provide uniformity in clinical judgment, they cannot be blindly applied without considering basic assumptions, clinical hypotheses, available evidence, contextual conditions, and so forth. To mitigate the impact of such pervasive limitations of clinical judgments, a great dosage of philosophy-inspired reasoning may be helpful, i.e. an out-and-out clinical philosophy. It is therefore necessary for clinical philosophy to be in continuity with other philosophical fields (logic, ethics, semiotics, philosophy of science, epistemology, etc.), in order to be sensitive to epidemiological and clinical issues, and at the same time, to be aligned with the idiographic nature of health care. Indeed, not only deductive and inductive forms of reasoning contribute to making better clinical decisions: abduction may also be a key tool in cases where probabilities cannot accurately prognosticate a patient. This is particularly true, as we have seen, when the clinical decision involves the consideration of conjectures based on conditions of fundamental uncertainty rather than well-known and quantifiable (probabilistic) risk factors. Moreover, the appropriate way to communicate health risks and uncertainties within informed consent is also discussed. Patients' perception of risks and uncertainties and the ability to imagine future scenarios play a key role in creating proper grounding for good clinical communication and shared health-related decisions.

Although the quality of medical care and technology is evolving at a rapid rate, the importance of values in health care cannot be stressed enough. By distinguishing the epistemic and non-epistemic (ethical, political, social) function of values, I have clarified the normative facets of clinical knowledge, in particular those related to what philosophers of science call "inductive risk" (the decision of the threshold of acceptable rates for false positive and false negative results), and presented a proposal for a conceptual explication of the notion of clinical possibility. The main idea is that purely epistemic considerations are not enough to handle the complexity of clinical reasoning. We need also to consider the non-epistemic functions and consequences of values in health care without discharging, as social constructivists often do, the epistemic dimensions of clinical knowledge, objectivity, efficacy, and empirical confirmation.

In conclusion, correct modes of reasoning may promote a form of clinical reasoning that increases knowledge, mitigates uncertainty and support better values for mankind.

References

Berchialla, P., Chiffi, D., Valente, G., Voutilainen, A.: The power of meta-analysis: a challenge for evidence-based medicine. Eur. J. Philos. Sci. (forthcoming) (2020)

Fuller, J., Flores, L.J.: The Risk GP Model: the standard model of prediction in medicine. Stud. History Philos. Sci. Part C: Stud. History Philos. Biol. Biomed. Sci. **54**, 49–61 (2015)

Appendix
The Diagnosis of Covid-19 for "Patient 1" in Italy

Interview to Dr. Annalisa Malara by Daniele Chiffi.

1. *It has been a while since you diagnosed COVID-19 to "patient 1" in Italy. What have you learned from this event?*

Almost two months have passed since that day and, looking back at the turn of events, I cannot but feel relieved and satisfied by the decision to carry out the diagnostic swab for COVID-19. In an intensive care unit, the severity of patients' clinical pictures requires making important decisions at very short notice.

The work of an intensivist doctor, however, is always the work of a team. Every decision being made is the result of continuous group sharing and critical review, also involving other specialists. And it is this work that makes the therapeutic process sounder whilst providing a continual professional growth. Our profession requires dedication and rigor, sacrifice and the awareness of the great responsibility we have. This can happen only if we keep in mind the central role of the patient. Thanks to the scrupulous and firm actions we made through collaborative team-work, and especially thanks to the fact that we did not rule out any possible aetiology, we could provide the patient with the best diagnostic-therapeutic chances, thus avoiding many other persons being exposed to the infection.

2. *Can you explain how you came up with your diagnostic hypothesis and, more generally, the structure and logic of your clinical reasoning?*

In an intensive care unit, you are faced with the most extreme clinical conditions, which often require a transversal methodological approach and an analogical thinking ability.

The severely affected clinical condition shown by the patient required impeccable diagnostic rigor: no hypothesis, however far-fetched, could be dismissed beforehand. The possible aetiology of coronavirus, presumed by the radiological and clinical characteristics of pneumonia, represented a true and unavoidable diagnostic possibility without which the patient's classification would have been shamefully incomplete. Plus, we could not ignore the connection with China, even if weak,

D. Chiffi, *Clinical Reasoning: Knowledge, Uncertainty, and Values in Health Care*, Studies in Applied Philosophy, Epistemology and Rational Ethics 58, https://doi.org/10.1007/978-3-030-59094-9

provided by the patient's wife. In approaching a disease, you have to search for all possible hypotheses; protocols therefore provide a skeleton on which to build clinical reasoning.

3. *Can you describe in detail how the clinical protocol for alleged patients with COVID-19 was structured before your diagnosis of "patient 1"? What intrinsic limitations did the application of the protocol contain that led you to violate it?*

As of 20/2, according to the protocol a patient was to be considered at risk of coronavirus infection only if he came from China or came into contact with people affected by coronavirus. The protocol in force on that date, in fact, did not prevent me from carrying out the examination in question; however, it would have justified a non-execution of the same examination since it was not deemed mandatory for the specific case.

4. *You said that because the known failed, you thought of the unknown. Do you want to clarify what you meant? What is the role of uncertainty in clinical practice?*

When faced with complex situations, linear thinking may not be enough. With the exception of frequent causes, when the most common therapies are not effective, we must consider even what seems more unlikely, yet still plausible. It is especially in the uncertainty of the diagnosis, of the therapy, and of the result, that you cannot underestimate anything.

5. *You have been called "the doctor who changed the life of all Italians". What ethical consequences do you think derive from taking such a bold diagnostic decision?*

When making a clinical decision, theoretical competence must go hand in hand with intuitive and deductive elements along with determination and responsibility in evaluating and deciding about the specific case.

That first diagnosis made it possible for an alarm to be raised in Italy and all throughout Europe; this led to subsequently obtain essential information on the asymptomatic transmission of the virus, and finally to provide precious time for implementing all containment measures designed to protect a very large number of people.

The case of Codogno is an example of an excellent way of working and reacting of the whole Italian Healthcare System, which has always been able to respond with professionalism and dedication to the public health needs of its citizens. Italian people, on their part, have traditionally been able to demonstrate outstanding intuition, tenacity, and resilience, even during particularly critical times.

The core principles of our profession are team-working with passion and dedication, by always maintaining the centrality of the patient; and it is thanks to such principles that we can bring health not just to our patients, but, in certain cases, to the whole community.

Printed in the United States
by Baker & Taylor Publisher Services